Throw out the negative programming from culture about weight loss, body shaming, and career dieting. *The Body Revelation* brings the true transformation we need. I trust no one more than Alisa Keeton to bring this solid word and get us moving in the right direction.

    LISA WHITTLE, bestselling author, speaker, and podcast host

Only Alisa could take the topic of pain and turn it into a triumphant message of motivation and movement—in every sense of the word. Inside these pages, you'll be moved by both her love for the Lord and her insight into how God designed our bodies. This isn't just a book to read; it's a book to practice.

    MICHELLE MYERS, cofounder of She Works His Way and author of the Conversational Commentary series

Ever wondered why you can't "just do it" when it comes to a healthy lifestyle? Or why your hard-fought results don't seem to last? Alisa Keeton knows exactly how you feel—and in *The Body Revelation*, she serves up proven solutions. With a motivating blend of scientific research, biblical wisdom, and true-life stories (plus super practical action steps at the end of each chapter), *The Body Revelation* is not just a good book to read. It actually has the power to be the best book you will ever *do*.

    JODIE BERNDT, bestselling author of *Praying the Scriptures for Your Life*

I've said for a long time that what happens in our souls, happens in our cells. We're fearfully and wonderfully made by the God who loves us! If you're ready to dig in, face your fears, and activate your faith, you're ready for *The Body Revelation*. Renewal and restoration await those who read slowly and prayerfully and are willing to apply what they've learned. Alisa Keeton is far more than a fitness expert; she's a healing and wholeness expert, biblically grounded and profoundly insightful. Having worked in the fitness industry for over a decade, I must say that she's one of the most balanced and biblical leaders out there. I loved this book.

    SUSIE LARSON, bestselling author, talk radio host, and national speaker

This book! Oh, the convergence of heart, soul, and body—in the form of a sage friend to hold our hand and speak into the things that lie underneath our skin and yet have so much power over our walk with God and the way we see the world. In this satisfying read, Alisa Keeton is our sage friend, gently inviting us into a new way of seeing God's heart and our bodies, and how they intersect. I'm so grateful for this message that Alisa carries with such passion.

SARA HAGERTY, bestselling author of *Unseen* and *Adore*

With so many bad messages about our good bodies floating around, I'm grateful for Alisa's voice in the world. *The Body Revelation* is informative, practical, and a huge source of encouragement. You can almost audibly hear her cheering you on through every page.

JJ HELLER, singer-songwriter

As a psychotherapist, I am captivated by the mind-heart-body connection. As Alisa brilliantly articulates, it's not simply diet and exercise that lead to health and healing. It's understanding how your story has shaped your wounds and led you to protect yourself in understandable yet unhelpful ways. *The Body Revelation* contains a wealth of wisdom, grounded in spiritual truth, that informs principles and practices that will not simply change your body but change your life. This is not a book to simply read. This is a book to practice—because it's in the practice that we are changed. I am personally grateful for Alisa's courage, vulnerability, and leadership. I know you will be too.

NICOLE ZASOWSKI, licensed marriage and family therapist and author of *What If It's Wonderful?*

The Body Revelation looks like a book, but it feels like a workout—a really good workout. This book is not hard to read, but it will be hard to forget. Alisa blends and stirs together a rich combination of stories, insights, information, and application. This book is a good meal and a great workout. It will stir your desire, your appetite, and your hope for things that are deep, real, and good in your heart, mind, and body. This kind of transformation is what people are seeking, searching for in therapy. We have seen, firsthand, the trajectory of people's lives changed. She writes like a good but dangerous friend. She extends a compelling and disruptive invitation to work out and work through our personal history, our real hurts, and our best hopes. It is a beautiful invitation.

DR. DON AND RENEE WORCESTER, therapist and spiritual coach, speakers, and ministry leaders

Alisa Keeton is a gift to this generation and a much-needed voice to the church. For too long in the West we have separated the heart and mind from the body, and it has caused us to miss out on the healing and deep intimacy the Lord has for us. This book is a game changer with deep insight and vulnerable stories. This is not a "feel good in your body" book but rather a liturgy of how we can grow deeper with Jesus by welcoming our bodies into the story. There's something about moving our bodies while rehearsing the truth of God's Word that transforms us. Alisa goes before us and walks with us as a teacher, preacher, and trainer in becoming formed more into the image of God.

ALYSSA BETHKE, author of *Satisfied*

No one in my life has encouraged me more in my journey with my body than Alisa. She has continually pointed me to the things that are true about my body and the One who created it. She has helped me see that God created me as a whole person—body, mind, spirit—and that all three need my attention. This book is one you will want to pass around to all your friends. Take in each chapter slowly and allow your thoughts to marinate in it. New patterns will develop. New kind words will be said to yourself by yourself! New mindsets will be created. I want this book to get into the hands of every woman who has ever—or will ever—think her body is bad.

JAMIE IVEY, bestselling author and host of *The Happy Hour with Jamie Ivey* podcast

The Body Revelation

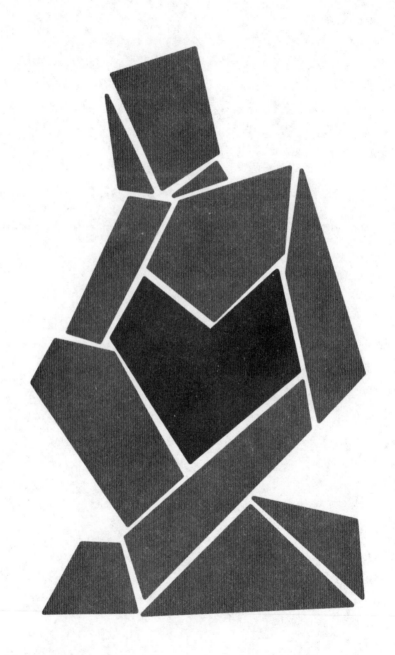

ALISA KEETON

The Body Revelation

Physical and Spiritual Practices to Metabolize Pain,
Banish Shame, and Connect to God with Your Whole Self

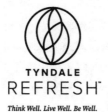

TYNDALE
REFRESH™

Think Well. Live Well. Be Well.

Visit Tyndale online at tyndale.com.

The Body Revelation: Physical and Spiritual Practices to Metabolize Pain, Banish Shame, and Connect to God with Your Whole Self

Published in association with Tawny Johnson of Illuminate Literary Agency: www.illuminateliterary.com

The stories in this book are about real people and real events, but names have been changed and some details changed to protect the privacy of people involved.

For information about special discounts for bulk purchases, please contact Tyndale House Publishers at csresponse@tyndale.com, or call 1-855-277-9400.

Library of Congress Cataloging-in-Publication Data

A catalog record for this book is available from the Library of Congress.

ISBN 978-1-4964-6260-2

Printed in the United States of America

29 28 27 26 25 24 23
7   6   5   4   3   2   1

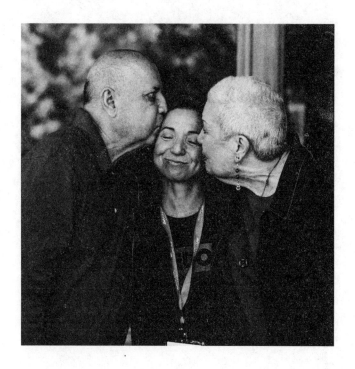

To my mama: A woman who lived with so much pain while here on earth but who now dances with Jesus and moves freely. Because of your story and love for Jesus, others will read this book and be set free.

To my dad: A complicated man whose need for Jesus led our family to Jesus and whose prayers I know I stand on today.

You both now live a life in heaven that your pain made hard to live on earth.

This book is for you.

CONTENTS

The Cooldown

FOREWORD

My story with Alisa is one for the ages.

I've played it back a million times to make sure I'm not exaggerating, and here are the broad strokes:

I was a woman who desperately needed wisdom about my body. What I thought I wanted was to lose weight; what I needed was truth and healing. I thought I wanted to change my life by changing my body; Jesus wanted to redeem my life by mending my relationship with my body. And in a move that I can only imagine was led by the Holy Spirit, I sent Alisa (who was no more than an acquaintance at the time) an email in the middle of the night asking for help. She responded the next day.

Alisa immediately informed me that while she would not promise to give me what I wanted, she'd be faithful to walk with me as God gave me what I needed. And the rest is history.

She coached me, corrected me, taught me, challenged me—all with large doses of love and compassion. And there was no going backward after that: The freedom train was rolling, the Spirit of God took over, and before I knew it, I loved my body more, I loved God more, and I was more keenly aware of just how loved I was.

I don't know why you picked up this book. Maybe you want to lose weight, maybe you are sick of being sick. Perhaps the persistent pain in your life has you at the breaking point, or you may just be curious about the intersection of faith and your body.

Here's my warning: Buckle up. Stay present. Keep going. You are safe, even if you feel that your shame and pain are very much in danger of defeating you.

Alisa is still the kind, wise, compassionate guide that she was for me. Maybe you've tried—maybe you've even had some success at—making healthier choices but still feel stuck. Alisa will show you how to partner with your body to begin processing the pain that has kept you trapped. She will teach you how to move your body and quiet your mind in ways that will bring lasting healing and better health. God *is* going to use this book to change your life.

Alisa has structured *The Body Revelation* around the typical parts of a Revelation Wellness training session. Come curious for the warm-up, enjoy going all in during the workout, and then watch God seal in life change during the cooldown. You're never going to be the same again, though it might not be in the ways you expect.

Your body is a revelation of Kingdom proportion, and God is going to reveal Himself to you right where you're at . . . in the good body you're in.

Trust me, this book is for you. It's for me too.

Your friend in the fight,

JESS CONNOLLY

Author of *Breaking Free from Body Shame* and *You Are the Girl for the Job*

INTRODUCTION

Moving the Bad Out of Your Good Body

SOME NIGHTS MY FATHER DIDN'T COME HOME.

The next evening, dinner would be tense. For long minutes, the scratching of metal forks and knives against porcelain plates was the only sound. I kept my head down, feeling the icy chill from the cold shoulder my mom was giving my dad.

He was determined to pretend that all was well. "Hey, honey, did I tell you I'm going to have to travel again next week for work?"

I slunk in my chair, seething with quiet rage. I would eat a hunk of Mom's casserole as fast as possible so I could run out the door and hop on the banana seat of my sunflower yellow, one-speed bike.

When I was a child, the sense of feeling small, unheard, and unseen in my family always seemed to dissipate when I went outside and moved my body. Moving made me feel big, free, and full of possibilities. It also allowed me to forget about how much my parents fought. I would pop wheelies on my bike or roller-skate like a disco queen, and somehow that just made me feel better.

By the time I was a teenager, any illusion I had of coming from a happy home with two parents who madly loved each other and laughed with their children at dinnertime was disappearing. When I needed a hug, I received a lecture. When I needed to be heard, I was asked to do the dishes. When I needed to be celebrated just for being me, I was told to clean my room.

Disappointment, loneliness, and sadness burned deep inside me like a fire, and angry outbursts were my only release. Some people choose to keep their feelings swept under the rug, and some people, like me, choose to light the rug on fire.

Then at fourteen, I attended my first group aerobics class with my friend Julie. I laced up a pair of white Keds, threw on my favorite T-shirt and some stinky gym shorts, and headed for Fitness Source, the gym at a nearby strip mall.

That initial workout seemed like choreographed chaos to me, but during cooldown I lay very still on the brown carpet as an incredibly warm feeling of comfort and peace washed over me. I had never felt this feeling before. Not with this intensity. It went beyond the feeling of freedom I had when I rode my bike or skated through the neighborhood. My eyes pooled with tears as I lay there gently stretching and wondered, *What just happened?* Perhaps it was the endorphin rush after shimmying and shaking for an hour in a crowd of middle-aged moms, or maybe it was simply pent-up teenage energy looking for a release. But whatever it was, at that moment I had the profound sense of hope dislodging my anger and sadness. I could feel it in my bones. It was as if something deep inside my body was telling me everything was going to be all right.

Whatever brought it on, I was hooked. With money from babysitting, I purchased my first pair of Reebok aerobic high-tops, bought the hot pink spandex leotard with matching belt (which I never understood, since it's not as if a tight leotard has a fighting chance of falling down), and paid the monthly dues to secure my place on a 1,500-square-foot of brown carpet with a record player in the corner. For just an hour a week, in a room filled with moms sporting colorful 80s makeup and crimped hair in scrunchies, I found a place I could call my own. For a teenage girl trying to figure out who she was, what she wanted, and where she was going, it was there I first felt safe to work these things out. It was there I began to experience a deeper connection between my heartache and my moving body. It was there I felt empowered in my own skin. I learned how to harness the fire of my teenage angst with a good calorie burn while feeling a sense of belonging. Instead of trying to tiptoe on eggshells around my mom's emotional outbursts and parents' exacting standards, here I could fumble freely, fall, or even step out of sync with the others and not be scolded. Mistakes were expected and trying again was celebrated.

My passion for learning how to move my body and gain strength—while feeling a sense of emotional relief—continued to grow. As a college sophomore, I spotted a flyer in the student union about a class on becoming a group fitness instructor. If I could help other people feel as safe and empowered in relationship to their bodies through fitness as I had become, I knew I had found my calling. By the time I graduated from college, I had a waiting list of clients who wanted to work with me. And because of that, I felt "loved," sought out, and wanted. I was truly living my dream. I was sure I'd moved far, far away from my dysfunctional home life—plus I was helping others!

When a fitness trainer I worked with told me she thought I'd be a real contender in fitness shows, I began bodybuilding, hoping I'd finally discovered the key to filling the void inside me. Before long, I was bringing home trophies. On the outside, I appeared to have it all together—more money than my fellow graduates who hustled in their nine-to-five, plenty of recognition and awards for a killer physique. But deep inside, my dissatisfaction continued to build.

Despite my parents' poor track record, I thought a romantic relationship might heal my aching heart. Yet almost every one of my boyfriends came and went, telling me "I just don't think I can give you what you want" as they broke things off. Then at twenty-six, I got married. I covered my pain in a white wedding dress and walked down the aisle and into the arms of an unsuspecting man.

I married Simon expecting that the love and commitment of one person would heal my hurts and quench the fire that burned within me. Instead, I quickly realized that nothing exposed my chronic dissatisfaction more than marriage. My husband's desire to climb the corporate ladder kicked into overdrive right after our wedding. Instead of candlelight dinners followed by snuggling with him while watching movies on the couch, I was home alone. And when he was home, Simon was a man of few words or—more accurately—a man of no words who had nothing left to give me after a long day at work. My growing discontentment fueled my expectations even more. And like a woman going to an empty well, I kept demanding more from Simon than he was able to give. My irrational emotional out-bursts and my tendency to give my husband the cold shoulder in our warm bed was starting to feel painfully familiar. Turns out, the pain of my childhood—feeling unwanted by an unfaithful father, unseen by a mother with fragile emotions, and unheard in a household with no room for my voice—threatened my longing for the family of my dreams.

The family I never had.

And there was no way I was going to fail at that like my parents did.

As a fitness professional in pursuit of good health, I knew something deep inside me was sick and needed help. My soul was crying out for the unconditional love and attention I lacked in my youth. For years I had done everything I could think of to push past the pain I'd grown up with. I'd tried to sweat it out, romance it out, and reason it out. Nothing worked.

Getting Unstuck: Moving from the Inside Out

Then God showed up—or rather I did. I'd heard about Him, of course, but I hadn't given Him much thought until my friend Shawn challenged me to attend the church where she'd recently met God. After some resistance, I went. I was so desperate and my heart so brittle and broken that I allowed Jesus, the Living Water, to seep in. He was coming to me in my pain but had no intention of leaving me there. God was about to turn everything I knew about fitness upside down and inside out. He understood that I needed more than simply changing the shape of my body or taking another lap around the gym. He knew a daily walk of faith with Him would restore my heart.

But He wasn't going to toss my love for movement aside. I had no idea that when I placed my trust in Jesus, I gave Him not only my heart, but my mind and body too. My first book, *The Wellness Revelation*, taught people how to look at their pursuit of good health holistically with God at the center. Readers were encouraged to consider how their relationship with God affected their relationship to themselves, other people, and other created things—like food.

After that book came out, I had conversations with many community and faith leaders. As a way of affirming my message that in Christ we are able to live a healthy and whole life, some well-intentioned people quoted 1 Corinthians 6:19-20: "Do you not know that your body is a temple of the Holy Spirit within you, whom you have from God? You are not your own, for you were bought with a price. So glorify God in your body." While I love this passage, I noticed that it was often stated like a Christian version of the Nike slogan "Just do it!" with little love or understanding for those who habitually struggle to adopt a healthy lifestyle. Yes, it's true; we are called to honor God with our bodies. But wouldn't we agree that if people could "just do it," they would have done it by now? It's not as if anybody wants to stay sick or stuck in a cycle of trying and failing. Heavy expectations are the last thing people need when they know they are falling short.

While *The Wellness Revelation* helped many people, it made me aware that it is possible to believe in God and either do all the right things or not do any of them and still feel stuck. The root cause of such disintegrated living needs to be identified and dealt with. I suggest that the absence of change and distance from God may not be due to a lack of willpower or love for Him but to our lack of awareness of how pain has disrupted our body-brain connection.

Years ago God let me in on a secret—how the bodies He's given us are useful for metabolizing, not just food, but also mental and emotional pain. God's view of health and fitness includes partnering with the natural healing processes of our body, activated through physical activity, God's Word, and spiritual practices, to metabolize pain. In *The Body Revelation*, we'll discover how to harness our bodies' natural healing properties and access tools to help us overcome rather than be overwhelmed by adversity. By maintaining a strong body-brain connection during adverse moments, the hurtful experiences of the past and the challenging moments in our future can be used as actual fuel—the energy we need—to live the lives God destined for us.

This book is less about finding the right eating plan and doing the right workout and more about doing the patient and kind work of becoming aware of the pain that disrupts a healthy body-brain connection and keeps us cycling in an unhealthy pattern of obsessing over or neglecting our bodies. By applying God's Word to physical and spiritual practices, we can renew our minds and live fully connected to ourselves for the purpose of moving toward the promise and purpose God has for us.

Please note: *The Body Revelation* is designed to start you on a journey toward health and wholeness, but it is not intended as a substitute for medical advice. It's important to talk with your own physician if you plan to make significant changes to your diet and exercise routines. Also, if you're looking for a quick fix, this isn't the book for you. We will be patient and kind with ourselves because that's what love does. And it's the love of God that changes everything!

Working the Plan

By the end of this book, you will stop trying to change yourself into a better version of you. You will know how to partner with your body to maintain peace by staying connected to yourself and God. As you learn to metabolize your pain, using movement and gospel-centered self-care spiritual practices that incorporate and activate God's Word, you will encounter through your body the God who loves you, knows you, and wants only the best for you. His love will change you, slowly and steadily, because slow and steady is the way to all sustainable change. And when hard moments come, you will overcome rather than be overwhelmed so you can stay free to become the person God created you to be.

Slow and steady is the way to all sustainable change.

While doing this work of reintegration, it's important that you feel safe. And one way safety occurs is through a plan. Every safe and effective class works through three phases: the warm-up, the workout, and—the best part (if you ask me)—the cooldown. Each phase of our workout time together will include two goals broken into two stages, all designed to help us metabolize the pain our bodies are holding. Here's what our workout will look like:

The Warm-Up
Stage 1: Just Surviving
Stage 2: Recognizing Your Pain

The Workout
Stage 3: Expressing Your Energy
Stage 4: Humbling Yourself

The Cooldown
Stage 5: Staying the Course
Stage 6: Taking Ownership

Each stage includes four bite-sized, digestible chapters concluding with a reflective, self-care section titled "Metabolize." Please don't skip this section. It's one thing to read and get useful information, but knowledge alone doesn't change a person. It's acting on that information that rewires a broken body-brain connection. It's doing new things that brings about internal and external change.

Each Metabolize section includes Mind, Mouth, and Move subsections. You will be asked to use your mind to answer a few questions related to that chapter. You will then use your mouth to pray and connect to God. Finally, I will invite you to engage in some healthy habits and doable physical movement to help you connect your thoughts and feelings about the things of God with your body. These Mind, Mouth, and Move sections are very important to making real body-brain connected change.

Moving your body is a critical part of metabolizing your pain. As I've worked with countless students over the years, I've seen that when our bodies move, our minds seem to receive God's Word with less resistance. I've lost count of the breakthrough aha moments that have occurred for my students while moving their bodies over the years. Here's how I think this works: Physical exercise engages the limbic system in our brain, which is where our instinctual flight, fight, or freeze response occurs. With the limbic brain productively occupied, higher reasoning seems to occur more easily.[1] In addition, the increase in oxygenated blood flow helps us think more clearly and boosts our mood. All of this makes it easier to access and process thoughts and feelings that have felt stuck in our body, keeping us trapped in poor habit loops.

Our bodies are how love makes its way into the world. More than building muscles and minimizing fat, we need bodies that are fit to carry love to others; for example, by carrying groceries up a flight of stairs to a single mom in need or by being rested and mentally sharp enough to patiently help our kids with their homework. In this book we will train to love God, ourselves, and others—all of which glorify God. His love holds all things together, mobilizes us to love in word and deed, and is the core strength of a healthy mind-body connection.

At its heart, this is a fitness and wellness book, written by me with guidance from the Holy Spirit, with one goal in mind: to bring freedom to captives of pain. Please don't skip the sweaty parts. Because I know that many of you will encounter a radical change in how you feel when moving your body with this new perspective, you may want more ways to move while renewing your mind with God's Word. At the back of the book you will find additional links to workouts and resources from Revelation Wellness, the nonprofit ministry I founded in 2011. Fitness and wellness are our ways of spreading the Good News of God's love to good bodies around the world. If you're looking for a coach to lead you through this book or a small group to go through the book with, be sure to check our website to find a Revelation Wellness instructor near you.

Don't just read this book. Do this book! Read, then join me in the training to metabolize your pain. I will be with you every step of the way. God has designed a wonderful life for you that lies just beyond the boundaries of your pain.

So let's train!

The Warm-Up

Just Surviving

There was a man who had two sons. And the younger of them said to his father, "Father, give me the share of property that is coming to me." And he divided his property between them.

LUKE 15:11-12

CHAPTER 1

THE FIRE OF YOUR DESIRE

Up and down the stairs she went.

It was a sight I had never seen before. Whenever I came home from school, I could count on finding my mom working hard somewhere around the house. Whether she was feverishly ironing our clothes with a can of spray starch clutched in her hand or scrubbing the cold Spanish floor tiles on her hands and knees with a bucket of Pine-Sol, she was always working hard at something. It was Mom's way of surviving another day.

But this type of hard work was a new sight for my seven-year-old eyes. Why was Mom sweating so heavily and breathing so hard, going up the stairs and coming right back down? She didn't even have a load of laundry in her hands! Then it clicked—my mom was exercising! Gasp! She was willingly subjecting herself to physical work that had no benefit to our family as cleaning the house or preparing a meal would.

This was 1978, and moving our bodies wasn't at the forefront of people's minds like it is now. The days of wearing yoga pants in public and purchasing green juice concoctions at the mall were in the distant future. But thanks to a few sweatband- and stretchy pants–wearing pioneers like Jack LaLanne and Richard Simmons, the message of reshaping the human body was beginning to take hold. The methods were simple: diet, exercise, and the calories-in-calories-out formula. It certainly had grabbed the attention of my thirty-year-old mom, who wanted her twenty-year-old body back.

Then one day a couple of months later, it all stopped.

Maybe Mom hung up her sneakers after another screaming blowout with my dad or maybe it was another morning when she woke up to realize that her husband hadn't come home the night before. Mom's continual disappointment with her husband, the man who was supposed to love and cherish her, was depleting her energy, reinforcing the lies of her youth, and overpowering any hope for change. Mom hadn't been caring for her body as an act of kindness toward herself. Her only motivation had been to whip her body into shape in hopes of regaining my father's love.

Each time she woke up in the middle of the night to find the other side of the bed empty, the message of being unchosen, unworthy, and unattractive grew stronger. *You're worthless; just give it all up already.* Taking control of her post-baby body was not enough to hold my father's affections. She must have decided, Why bother? And just like so many other women who wake from their fairytale dream of someone rescuing them from their destitute castle of pain, my mom had woken to the nightmare of dashed hopes and unmet desires.

Over the years I watched my mom physically shut down. She traded in burning calories by running up and down the stairs to more bingeing of calorie-laden foods. Food numbed her pain and became her comfort, her go-to friend. It was the early 1980s and the processed food industry was in high gear. Packaged goodies, potato chips, and TV dinners promised pleasure and convenience. This revolution in ready-to-eat food made "friends" available to her in the pantry, at the corner fast-food joint, convenience store, and nearly everywhere she went.

It was as if Mom slowly began to build a barricade around her body with food. She used it to insulate herself from the emotional pain of the world and the physical touch of my father.

The weight of her disappointment started in her heart, unseen, but eventually made its way onto her body to be seen and judged by all. Each excess pound compounded the message of shame she already carried in her heart, making it harder for her to move and breathe deeply.

Why Pain Must Be Processed

My mom was stuck, but she was safe. Surviving and safe.

You can't bury or evict hurt and suffering; it must be metabolized or, to put it another way, processed. I define pain as any life experience that made you feel bad, sad, mad, or scared and that, whether you know it or not, has left a lasting negative effect on you. Let me ask you a question: What if a bad experience you suffered, childhood neglect you endured, shame you carry, or hurtful words you absorbed not only got stuck in your head but in your body too? Your body has been with you through all the hard times, sorting, filing, and storing the energy of your pain in order to help you live through another day. And although your body is efficient at internalizing your pain, it isn't efficient in actually dealing with it.

You can't bury or evict pain; it must be metabolized.

Research shows that when the brain receives information combined with a negative emotional charge—as when a loved one dies, someone you love's been hurt, or someone you love hurts you—your nervous system can become overwhelmed.[1] This is known as a trauma response, and in these moments, the body-mind connection that usually helps you purposely move through life stops working optimally. Instead, it simply tries to help you survive the moment and stay safe. Bessel van der Kolk, MD, respected trauma researcher and author of the bestselling book *The Body Keeps the Score*, says, "Traumatized people chronically feel unsafe inside their bodies: The past is alive in the form of gnawing interior discomfort. Their bodies are constantly bombarded by visceral warning signs, and, in an attempt to control these processes, they often become expert at ignoring their gut feelings and in numbing awareness of what is played out inside. They learn to hide from their selves."[2]

In essence, your body can feel more like an enemy than a friend since it becomes the storage room for your pain. Whether you lived through adversity when you were five or thirty-five, you experienced these upsetting moments, not just emotionally or cognitively, but with your whole body, your whole self.[3] This "bad stuff" stuck in your good body is not your fault, and it can be moved out. In this book we are going to move it out together.

Pain from your past may be getting in the way of healthy living for you if you find yourself:

1. blaming others when anything bad happens to you
2. harboring unresolved shame
3. assuming you are the problem in every situation

Each of these actions can help you feel safe, but hiding out in these go-to emotional shelters can never free you to be who God made you to be. I should know: I was once the reigning queen of assigning blame. It was a way of projecting my pain onto someone else. But the weight of criticizing everyone else became far too heavy a burden for me to carry. Yes, like my mom, I learned it could keep me feeling safe and in control, but it always backfired and pushed me further from the true love—unconditional, patient, and kind—that I longed for.

Mom lived with one primary desire burning inside of her. It's a desire we all share—to be loved. Our hunger to be loved includes the need to be seen, heard, valued, and chosen. We all look for someone who is committed to being faithful to us in sickness and in health, in good times and bad times, until death do we part.

When it comes to that desire, I've got some good news and bad news.

First, the bad news: Our desire for love (to be seen, heard, valued, and chosen) will never be filled by another human being. Every person's love is temporal and will fail us, just as every weight-loss diet we've tried works for a while but can't be sustained forever.

Now the good news: This love we long for can be found in Jesus Christ. He is fully God and fully man, and He put on flesh and came to earth, not to condemn us but to rescue us from the endless search for the love we once had but lost.

Placing our faith in Jesus helps us put everything, including our desires, back in working order. He helps us determine whether our desires come from God or derive from our pain. According to Jeremiah 17:9, the human heart is "deceitful above all things . . . who can understand it?" God, the one who gave you a heart and a body, understands it. When we give Him our hearts' desires, He empowers us to break free from choices that drive present, past, and future pain.

When Desire Causes Pain

A desire, according to my dictionary, is a "conscious impulse toward something that promises enjoyment or satisfaction."[4]

At our core, each of us is a pleasure seeker because God is the author of pleasure. He seems to have hardwired a desire for enjoyment into each one of us so that we might find Him. In fact, desire, like hunger, is a very good thing. Satisfying both is necessary to our survival.

In the case of Adam and Eve, desire and hunger looked identical when a serpent came calling. These first two people, living as one, were in perfect relationship with God and creation until their desire for something that looked pleasing to their eyes and stomachs overpowered their devotion to God. Led away by a lie, they gave in to the desire for something pleasurable apart from Him.

When we desire things that God doesn't, we come to ruin:

> For many, of whom I have often told you and now tell you even
> with tears, walk as enemies of the cross of Christ. Their end is
> destruction, their god is their belly, and they glory in their shame,
> with minds set on earthly things.
>
> PHILIPPIANS 3:19-20

As a child, I saw this play out in my own family. My mom believed the lie that a man's love would bring her unending pleasure, while my father believed the lie that the love of many women would satisfy him. When God isn't the source of our pleasure, the one we look to determine our desires, we run into problems and bring pain to ourselves and others.

James 4:1 says, "What causes fights and quarrels among you? Don't they come from your desires that battle within you?" (NIV). According to James, it's not our lack of faith in God that causes problems among us; it's the desires we feel we must satisfy. Like my mom, who depended on a man to rid her of the rejection she felt as a child, we may carry around unmet desires, making unhealthy choices in an effort to satisfy our needs. My father did the same thing. Both my parents misplaced and misused desire.

When we misplace our desires, we look for them to be met by other people or things who may be unwilling or incapable of fulfilling those needs. And in the misuse of an unmet desire, we either express our pain by explosively unloading our disappointment onto others or we repress our feelings by burying them deep inside. We often are totally unaware of how the explosion or repression of our feelings affects other areas of our lives, including our physical health.

Author and mental health specialist Louise B. Miller points out that "losing your temper affects your cardiac health, it can shorten your life when sustained. Anger also compromises your immune system."[5] And a study from the University of Texas found that when we avoid expressing our emotions, we exhaust our self-control, which can actually strengthen our negative emotions in the future. This, in turn, can lead to many physical and mental maladies.[6]

Those are our unhealthy choices: Explode and oppress others, or do nothing and repress ourselves. Either way, everybody pays the price of pain due to misplaced desires. But there is a God-given way to fulfill desire: Instead of exploding or repressing, we can learn to take our hurts to God and process our unmet desires with Him. In this book you will learn how to put pain to good use as you discover ways to develop and maintain a strong body and brain connection, which will strengthen your faith and abiding love for God.

As we've said, desire isn't necessarily bad or a cause of pain. Desire is God-given and the way He uses us to bring more of His Kingdom to earth. We hope or desire for things like a great marriage, friendship and companionship, world peace, good health, clothes that fit, less stress, and even more likes on Instagram. None of these are destructive in themselves.

It's when what we want usurps our desire to know and enjoy God and to fulfill His commands that they become ungodly. Such desires are sinful (misplaced and misused), and they cause pain. Desiring to lose weight or gain muscle aren't bad things—it's when we expect these desires, once they are met, to satisfy us and give us what only God can that we can get or cause hurt. It's when we desire something more than God that our desires become destructive.

Desiring, seeking, and serving someone or something other than God is what the Bible calls idolatry. Idolatry fuels unmet, misplaced, and misused desires and contributes to physical sickness, weight loss, weight gain, disease, and dis-ease. Most tragically, idolatry results in disconnection from God, the Source of Life.

When Our Desire Causes God Pain

Throughout this book, we'll be returning to a story that Jesus told in an attempt to teach some tax collectors and sinners about God's Kingdom. This story centers on a wealthy father and his two sons, who seemed to have everything they could possibly need: a nice home with a warm bed and three square meals a day; important jobs working for the family business; seats of honor at the lavish parties their father threw. But the younger son's desire to explore the world outside his father's gates was so strong that it caused him to do a scandalous thing. He asked his father for his inheritance before his father's death: "Father, give me the share of property that is coming to me" (Luke 15:12). That was the equivalent of saying, "Father, you're dead to me."

How does a young man who seemingly had it all decide that life could be even better? Was this son more interested in life in the big city than on the farm? Was he suffering from a severe case of the grass is always greener? Or had he made friends with people who appeared to live more footloose and fancy-free? Did these friends give him a hard time and try to make him feel less than for having more? Or did this son always battle with a deep-seated root of insecurity that kept him from feeling satisfied with life? Jesus doesn't tell us the cause of this son's request, but we do know the effect. The younger son's desire to leave his father's presence grew so strong that he couldn't wait for his father to die. Just imagine the pain this must have caused his father's heart.

Before we judge this son too harshly, however, we must remember that we all suffer from the young son's condition because of the years we lived outside our Father's gates. Prior to putting our faith in God, we live as orphans on the earth, roaming the world looking for value, for something to "eat" to satisfy our inner ache. Our belief in God takes us off the streets and inside our Father's home and care. We are no longer orphans but chosen and adopted sons and daughters of a Father who lacks nothing and freely gives us all things.

We all come to God dragging a duffle bag filled with desires. These wants are everything that people outside our Father's gates tell us we should pursue—like the perfect body, the marriage of our dreams—and things we feel we must offer the world—like dazzling talents, skills, or abilities. If we leave this bag of desires unchecked at the door of our Father's house, we end up using them to decorate our room in our Father's house. We place these objects on our shelves like collectible figurines, reminding us daily of what we want our Father to give us.

Like the Prodigal Son, we cause pain to our Father's heart when we elevate things of this world above Him. When we think we can find life's enjoyment and satisfaction in other people, places, or things, we hurt God's heart. It's crazy to think we have the power to cause God pain, but if you've ever loved someone who didn't love you in return, you've experienced it too.

As we come back to the story of the Prodigal Son in later chapters, we'll consider what happened to him as he wandered away and what finally brought him home, back to the father whose heart was always full of love for his wondering-wandering child.

Our inability to desire and process pain in a healthy way can interfere, not only with our need for love, but with our ability to receive love. Needing implies a physical posture of grasping with our hands, while to receive, we must allow our hands to slacken and open. When we receive God's love, we soften our grip, stop striving, and drop our duffle bag. We entrust our lives fully to His care. Doing what He says feels like a delight, not a duty.

Many Christians say they love God from a posture of desiring protection and deliverance from their pain, but fewer love God because they have received His love with open hands, expecting healing from and transformation of their pain.

I'm about to say something that may sound provocative but is both biblical and true: God desires to love the hell out of us. He wants to expose and evict the dark places inside us—fear, shame, guilt, rejection, condemnation, insecurities, gluttony, pride, sexual immorality, selfishness, and greed. These are not in line with God's nature, character, or His Word, so they no longer need to be part of our reality. They lead to wrong desires that hurt us and cause more pain. But when we choose God, we choose His perfect, refining love. God's desire is to transform us until there's nothing left but His love with breath, bones, and muscle, covered in skin. Once He clears out the dangerous desires we carry inside of us, we are free to become the people we were meant to be.

> There is no fear in love. But perfect love drives out fear because fear has to do with punishment. The one who fears is not made perfect in love.
>
> 1 JOHN 4:18, NIV

God's love is not meant to just be a theology for our mind; it's meant to penetrate every cell of our being. With our renewed mind and joy-filled bodies, we are empowered to share His love with others. Our theology should influence our biology until we have a great biography—a story that glorifies our God who makes all things new.

Our theology should influence our biology until we have a great biography.

The only thing that can heal us, teach us, and empower us to change is God's love. In Christ, we are new creations. We are empowered by God's Spirit living inside of us to walk away from our old nature and unhealthy, co-dependent desires. We are free to stop dragging around our duffle bag of desires, filled with everything the world tells us we deserve or need, whether another sleeve of Oreo cookies, a bottle of wine, or six-pack abs and a flat stomach.

It's possible to love God but never let His love truly change us. For the sake of God's goodness, let Jesus love the pain, hurt, and shame out of you. That's what this book is here to help you to do! Admittedly, trying to make changes for the better, especially when it comes to health, is never easy. In fact, it can be downright crazy-making. The adversity you've experienced has negatively affected your brain's health, making it difficult to think clearly with your mind, stay hopeful in your heart, and make better choices for your body—like whether to take your body to the pantry for a snack or take it on a walk around the block and talk with God.

It's possible to love God but
never let His love truly change us.

My mom never learned what to do with her unmet desires and disappointments. She never learned how to partner her body of hurt with God's grace to be transformed into a new creation. Instead, with Jesus buried in her heart, she set up camp in the battleground of her pain, got stuck, and grew cold and bitter. But this doesn't have to happen to you.

That is why, though this book is designed to help you understand how pain affects your relationship with your body, we have no intention of remembering the hurt we've experienced in order to get stuck there. We will not replay the tapes of what was done, not done, or said over and over again in our heads. We will not glamorize, glorify, or build monuments to our pain. The goal instead is to learn how to stay present in your body and exercise the authority you have over it, by feeling what you feel, observing what you're thinking, and reorganizing that information until it supports your ability to move through life's pain checkpoints and into the life Christ died to give you.

You no longer have to remain in the pain of misplaced and unmet desires. You can release the bad stuff that's gotten stuck in your body. During my experience with thousands of students over the years, I've learned that getting unstuck from the dis-ease in our body isn't something we just need more faith for. A faith that moves us from surviving to thriving and living with purpose must be active or, according to James, it is not faith at all: "So then faith that doesn't involve action is phony." (James 2:17, TPT).

Be sure to do the work below to start metabolizing your pain. Soon you will be more able to think, feel, and choose in line with what God says is best for you.

Metabolize

Reading good information alone doesn't change a person. Only acting on that information will bring change to your body, brain, and life.

We will metabolize your pain using the three *M*s: Mind. Mouth. Move. The Mind section will help you think new things. The Mouth section is for you to declare and say a new thing. And the Move portion will ask you to do a new thing with your body. Thinking, saying, and doing are three essentials to trigger neuroplasticity—your brain's ability to adapt, change, and form new connections. Our goal is to strengthen healthy neural pathways, which will help bring vitality to your body. Improving your brain health while using your body as a tool is the method you will use to metabolize your pain.

Mind

1. What life desires leave you feeling chronically disappointed and cause you pain?
2. How has the pain of unmet desires affected your mind (thoughts), soul (what you desire), and body?
3. List some areas of pain in your life that could use Jesus' transforming love.

Mouth

In each chapter, please try praying the prayer out loud. The goal of this book is to embody faith. Use your vocal cords to let your ears hear what your heart desires to be true. Prayers don't have to feel real to be effective. Faith makes prayer effective, not our feelings.

God, my desires have brought me joy and distress. You have placed desires within me in order to bring good things into the earth, but I struggle to make these things happen without causing hurt to myself or others. I know I need to desire You more than anything or anyone else, but that idea seems foreign to me and if I'm honest, boring and unsatisfactory. Come and replace with your love anything that keeps me from desiring You. Help me to receive Your love until my mind, will, and emotions mirror You, for then my body will live in good health. Amen.

Move

Begin to move your body with the primary objective of processing your pain rather than changing the shape of your body. If you are able, get outside and go for a walk while listening to the short audio recording I designed for you. You will move your body at a moderate pace, feeling your blood flow and breathing rate increase as you listen to my voice coach you through some of the concepts you learned in this chapter (and chapters to follow). The goal is to get in your body by getting in touch with what your body is feeling physically and sensationally in order to process the pain and get unstuck.

Each Move recording is twenty minutes long. The goal is to appropriately challenge yourself with kind, mind-renewing movement, not an extreme calorie burn. If you're prone to obsess over your body's fitness level and always wear a fitness tracker, you may want to take it off. You're not trying to "crush" a workout. I want to get you back in your body in a gentle, curious, and kind way. If you've been neglecting your body and it's been a while since you've moved, don't be afraid if your breathing feels a little challenged, but also try to avoid pushing yourself to the point that you are breathless.

Whether or not you regularly exercise, this way of moving will likely be a totally new experience and a key step to begin processing your pain.

We are all in this together!

Find the link to the Move audio that goes with this chapter here: https://www.revelationwellness.org/tbr/move/.

If you find new joy in moving your body this way (which I am certain you will), be sure to access more kind, mind-renewing movement available to you on page 274.

CHAPTER 2

THE CALORIE BURN

"CALORIES IN, CALORIES OUT." It's a simple math equation, right? Maybe. I've known many men and women who could've earned a BCA (bachelor's degree in caloric accounting) from WLU (Weight Loss University) but still didn't get the results they were looking for from that formula.

There's now an app to count the calories in a tablespoon of ice cream or one square of a candy bar, so dieters always know how much to withdraw from their calorie bank account and how much remains. Yet despite all the fuss and time-consuming attention to detail, some people never see the change they hoped for or are unable to sustain a smaller waistline. Some people end up working full-time in what I call the Food Police Force, taking on the job of keeping bad foods behind bars.

The tit for tat; eat this, don't eat that is a losing game for us human beings. Our emotions go up and down as we categorize and count points. For those of us who find it difficult to feel our feelings and take agency over our lives, measuring and weighing may bring a sense of control. But if this meticulous pursuit could produce lasting change, you probably wouldn't be reading this book.

When it comes to our bodies and food, we need a bigger perspective. So let me share the bottom line: Your body needs energy to survive and thrive. All food is energy. Some energy burns longer and better than others.

If I were stranded on a desert island without food, I would not deny myself a box of doughnuts that washed up on shore, even though it's not the most nourishing food to eat. (I'm not sure how an intact box of dough-nuts would have made it to my island, but now you know my kryptonite when it comes to tempting food.) Everything we eat is a source of energy. Every person who lives, breathes, feels, thinks, and moves must consume energy to make it through the day.

With that in mind, as a formula for moving numbers on the scale, let's choose "energy in, energy out" rather than "calories in, calories out." We need energy to sustain life, but some sources of energy are better than others at upgrading and transforming our lives.

Choose "energy in, energy out"
rather than "calories in, calories out."

God designed life on earth to exist inside an energy ecosystem of input and output, receiving and giving, sowing and reaping, building up and tearing down. What goes in will come out. Without the desire to live for something greater than six-pack abs and money in the bank, the daily grind of consuming and expending energy feels good in the moment, but then we are left with the aftereffects of whatever we consumed. Eating for either comfort or vanity is futile and has fleeting results.

My mom used food for comfort; I used it more for vanity. I fell into this food trap when my simple enjoyment of fitness became my obsession. In my early twenties, I tucked the pain of my childhood away inside my gym bag. I used it as my hidden source of energy and headed for the fitness competition stage. Under bright lights, I was drowning in baby oil and showing off a sponge-on tan that had turned me the color of mahogany wood. I showed off my fit body—never mind that it was dehydrated and the growling sounds of my hunger pains went head to head with the nineties grunge music that played in the background. The trophies at my feet and medals around my neck were living proof that the energy I was spending made me a success.

Except for one thing: I was totally miserable. The fifteen minutes on stage were not worth the eight months of misery during training. Even though I wasn't walking with Christ back then, somehow I knew that all the time and energy I spent sculpting my body so I could stand on a stage to be scored and compared to other bodybuilding women was nothing but a vain pursuit. Exhausted by the endless pursuit of bodily perfection—a target that seemed to always be moving—I hung up my bikini and Lucite-heeled competition shoes after about five years. I was done trying to soothe my pain with the applause of people.

People who run from their pain often find comfort by living on a never-ending treadmill at high speed. As the belt of our days whizzes by underneath our feet, we grip the rails, jump and straddle the treadmill's belt, and catch our breath. We give ourselves just enough time to account for what we ate, what we did, or even stranger yet, what someone else ate or didn't do. Moving fast and keeping short tabs on ourselves and others may be effective for reaching our goals in the here and now but does nothing to gain what's eternal.

When a person made by God invites Him to be their source of energy—whether to improve their health, finances, or relationships—they trade in their high-paced treadmill (or Lucite heels) for a road and a pair of walking shoes. Life works best when we walk with God through the power and presence of His Holy Spirit.

Walk by the Spirit, and you will not gratify the desires of the flesh. For the desires of the flesh are against the Spirit, and the desires of the Spirit are against the flesh, for these are opposed to each other, to keep you from doing the things you want to do.
GALATIANS 5:16-17

As we journey with God, He slowly convinces us that we can't trust our flesh but we can trust Him. We can stop counting on all our physical tools—our food diaries, workout logs, measuring cups, and scales—and let Him lead. We can choose a slower pace—a thoughtful and kinder way. When it appears to the world that we are slowing down or getting soft, we are actually beginning to gain back what we lost—our souls.

> What good will it be for someone to gain the whole world,
> yet forfeit their soul? Or what can anyone give in exchange
> for their soul?
>
> MATTHEW 16:26, NIV

There is no amount of good energy we can take in or give out to gain back our souls. Only God wins them back and fills our hearts with His love so we can live and burn with His boundless energy.

Metabolism: The Great Exchange

Just as God's transforming love provides the energy we need to live peaceful and productive lives, so He designed a process within our bodies to change the food we consume into energy. Think of a fire inside a woodburning stove that requires hardwood logs to stay lit. That's a picture of metabolism: the chemical processes that occur within a living organism to maintain life.[1] Metabolism provides the energy needed to keep us alive and breathing.

Right now you are filled with and burning energy. You are lit! (Excuse the Gen Z pun.) Whether it's the burrito you ate for breakfast or stored muscle and fat, your body is burning something and turning it into chemicals for your body to use. Metabolism is like a party going on inside of you. Chemicals are dancing, bopping around, mingling, socializing, and exchanging hugs and handshakes. They mingle with other chemicals in your body to keep your eyes blinking, your throat swallowing, and your lungs breathing. Your chemical party is even making it possible for you to read this book right now. And some of those chemicals are party poopers who try to stop the fun (more on them later).

One cool fact about scientific processes is that a substance can change from one form into another. For example, burning paper turns into ash, a raw egg can be hard-boiled, milk can turn sour, and fruit can rot. What's also cool is that these processes can be studied and tested. In other words, a process of change can be proven.

We experience another type of change once we put our faith in Christ: "Therefore, if anyone is in Christ, the new creation has come: The old has gone, the new is here!" (2 Corinthians 5:17, NIV).

We can weigh our bodies and count calories in food, but the spiritual process that the apostle Paul writes about is harder to measure and see. Instead of a calorie exchange, we receive a character exchange. Something happens inside to plug us into a more excellent source of energy than ourselves. This source is God's love. When we know He loves us, our hearts come alive, and we are motivated to know His love more. As we do, we each begin to know our true self, the self that is free of fear, shame, or guilt. The self that is prone to stay stuck in pain. When a person begins to live without fear, shame, and guilt, that is a noticeable change! God is the one who makes us and knows us, inside-out, from our soul to our skin. Just as our body's metabolism converts food into energy, this character exchange process fuels our desire for new life and helps us live it out. And just like the chemical process of our body's metabolism, the change in our lives can be tested and proven.

Just as our body's metabolism converts food into energy, the Spirit's character exchange process fuels our desire for new life.

Notice the exchange we experience through God, which the apostle Paul describes in the following verses:

We do not lose heart. Though outwardly we are wasting away, yet inwardly we are being renewed day by day. For our light and momentary troubles are achieving for us an eternal glory that far outweighs them all.

2 CORINTHIANS 4:16-17, NIV

You have turned my mourning into dancing for me;
You have taken off my sackcloth and clothed me with joy.
PSALM 30:11, AMP

Those who sow in tears
shall reap with shouts of joy!
PSALM 126:5

In short, the metabolism of God's fire burns to exchange

- our old self for a new self;
- greater care and concern for our insides than our outside;
- lies that keep us stuck for truth that sets us free;
- mourning for what we have lost into dancing for what's been gained; and
- tears that bring healing into joy that brings life.

Our new metabolism is a work of God's Spirit living inside of us, walking with us and teaching us day after day. The Spirit in us changes us from the inside out. In Christ, we each have a revved-up, fired-up, never fading, always burning spiritual metabolism! It's fire! It's fierce! And it puts to shame all the thermogenic weight-loss supplements that tinker with chemical processes in our body.

The Energy of Faith

I am drawn to science because I have always been fascinated by how things work. Science guides us in studying and making sense of the world around us. Although some people try to separate science and faith, they actually fit together perfectly since God is the creator of *all* things. It's as if God placed curiosity and wonder inside all His children, hoping we will find Him when we are ready to have eyes of faith to see.

Faith picks up the slack when evidence-based science does not yet have permission from God to explain what is happening. What we don't have answers for, we can accept by faith.

Fact:[2] All matter contains energy.

Before the twentieth century, scientists assumed that all matter—the things we can touch, weigh, measure, and feel—could be seen. (We humans like to measure what we can observe and propose theories to help us make sense of what we don't understand.) The study of what we can measure and see is called Newtonian physics. For example, an object's movement stays the same unless something else changes it, and for every reaction there is an equal and opposite reaction. By the early twentieth century, scientists knew that the atom was the smallest known form of matter. However, they wanted to know the substance of an atom, so they split it.

Guess what they found when they split the atom? Atoms aren't made up of more matter. We currently depict the atom as protons and neutrons clustered together with electrons whizzing around them on the outside. And here's something very strange: Atoms are 99.9999999 percent empty space.[3]

Could this mean that the smallest part of us is the bigger part of us? That the smallest part of us (energy) drives and affects what we see as the more significant parts of us (matter)—what we can touch, taste, see and feel? Sounds a lot like faith to me! I suggest the intangible parts of you matter more to your health and to our God who is unseen than the tangible things that are seen. And it's the intangible God who is holding the seen and unseen things together:

> For by him all things were created, in heaven and on earth,
> visible and invisible, whether thrones or dominions or rulers or
> authorities—all things were created through him and for him.
> And he is before all things and in him all things hold together.
>
> COLOSSIANS 1:16-17

Everything made contains more of something we can't see than what we can see. In addition, the world is held together by unseen forces, such as gravity and electromagnetic fields. The unseen things are the sustaining and driving force of creation. It sounds pretty Kingdom on earth to me!

God's Word is true when it says:

We fix our eyes not on what is seen, but on what is unseen, since what is seen is temporary, but what is unseen is eternal.

2 CORINTHIANS 4:18, NIV

Now faith is confidence in what we hope for and assurance about what we do not see.

HEBREWS 11:1, NIV

Do you see that? Faith has everything to do with believing in what we *do not see*! And since there is more to us that is unseen than seen, more to us that is energy than matter, faith provides the best fuel for the metabolic fire blazing in our bodies. Faith in God—the Creator of all things. And this includes faith for life in our bodies too!

Of course, in a world of matter, we are prone to think that matter is all that matters. But things go wonky on earth whenever we put our trust in things that are not of God. The Bible calls this idolatry—trusting in things we make with our hands and devote ourselves to, seeking to gain some sense of control in a chaotic world. Idols eventually fail.

God knew we would disobey Him, putting our trust and energy in things that aren't of Him. Things we can see. Yet He went ahead and created everything, and Jesus made a way for us to come back to the God who created us and gives us energy for faith. Because of Jesus, we can stop aimlessly whizzing around like frantic particles of energy, running on treadmills and counting calories, prone to worry and fear about the shape of our thighs or the strength of our biceps.

God loves us from our soul to our skin, from the unseen to the seen. He fills our empty spaces—the ones we often try to fill with misplaced desires—with His love and energy.

Metabolize

Mind

1. How have God's love and energy changed you?
2. How does knowing you are more energy (unseen) than solid matter (seen) change how you consider the kind of energy you consume?

3. On a scale of 1–10 (1 being lowest, 10 being highest), what's your average energy level each day? How could living from faith improve your energy level and body health when it comes to your thoughts, feelings, and choices?

Mouth

God, I need Your help. I am exhausted from keeping accounts of people and things who have hurt me. I need Your love, Your saving energy. I invite You to come and fill all of me and my empty spaces with Your presence. Amen.

Move

Counting calories can feel like a sensible practice when we want to improve our body and health, but it doesn't make us wiser to our wants. Being mindful of what goes into our body and how it makes us feel is a kinder, wiser, and more sustainable way to bring physical change. When we become aware of what we eat and how it makes us feel, we become our body's advocate rather than its adversary or food police. During our training time together, you are invited to start tracking these details using the daily food journal template on page 276, or you can order the ninety-day *Revelation Wellness Food Journal* from your favorite bookseller. As I stated in the introduction, this isn't a book about what to eat or not to eat. I hope by the time you finish *The Body Revelation*, you will be more aware of how food makes you feel rather than worrying about what foods you should or shouldn't eat. All the Move practices to come in the following chapters will support this end goal.

Find the kind-mind renewing movement that goes along with this chapter at this link: https://www.revelationwellness.org/tbr/move/.

CHAPTER 3

GOD'S TRANSFORMING FIRE

I WAS NEVER A BIG FAN OF SCIENCE IN SCHOOL. It wasn't something I saw as particularly helpful for my future. I had no vision of myself in a white lab coat studying slides under a microscope. I didn't know what I wanted to be when I grew up, but I knew it wouldn't have anything to do with science. (Cue the sounds of God's laughter since fitness and exercise are a science.)

Yet back then, I was eager to take one science class: chemistry. I suspect that was due to the episodes of *The Muppet Show* in which the Muppet scientist would boil some bubbling green concoction in a big glass beaker. Suddenly he'd pour in a little pink liquid mixed with blue goop and . . . *BOOM!* Muppet hair flew everywhere. But nobody got hurt. (If nobody suffered when things explode, there would be no need to write this book.)

In my sophomore year of high school, I entered the laboratory with my white coat and goofy-looking goggles, ready to make magic potions. *What will it be?* I thought. *Slime? Perhaps some sort of combustible soda can experiment? Please let something explode!* My mad-scientist aspirations died when the teacher told us we would heat ice and watch it turn into steam. *Umm . . . excuse me. Boring! What's the big deal? I've done this in the microwave like a thousand times.*

The teacher was introducing us to the world of thermodynamics—the branch of physics dealing with heat and other forms of energy. We were starting with the first law of thermodynamics: " Energy can neither be created nor destroyed, only altered in form."[1]

If you are hoping to practice what you will learn in this book, you mustn't forget this truth: Energy cannot be created or destroyed; it will either be transformed (changed into something else) or transmitted (passed on to someone else).

Energy cannot be created or destroyed; it will either be transformed (changed into something else) or transmitted (passed on to someone else).

Emotions are comprised of energy. The word *emotion* comes from the Latin word *emovere*, which means "to move out."[2] In essence, emotions are energy in motion, making their way through our bodies and waiting to be harnessed by our muscles so our bodies can release them into the world.

If you're a sports fan or have attended a ball game, you've participated in the rise and fall of emotions and the display of emotional energy. If the team you want to win succeeds at a tie-breaking play, an uplifting emotion like joy floods your nervous system. In an instant you're on your feet, punching your hands into the air and perhaps opening your mouth wide as you activate your vocal chords with breath to shout and cheer. But if your team is losing, your emotionally embodied energy experience is just the opposite. You stay in your seat, furrow your brow, and clench your fists and teeth. If you jump to your feet, it's only to yell at the ref who made a bad call.

Some emotions uplift us to embody joy, like when your team is winning. Some emotions downshift us into a state of calm and peace, like when you sit and watch the waves on a beach. Others can be downright destructive to ourselves or to those around us, like the fury you feel toward your favorite team's rivals or the shame you suppress after you failed to make a play on the field. Emotional pain that affects the posture of our body is called embodied cognition.[3] A study done by Penn State University showed that negative moods adversely affect our immune system by increasing inflammation in our bodies,[4] and sustained inflammation impairs our immune system. (More to come on inflammation in chapter 10.) So not only does the energy of emotional pain affect the posture of our bodies, but it also can suppress our bodies' ability to fight off sickness and disease. Emotions are energy. They hold the power to uplift us or to discourage us—but either way, we will pass them on to others.

Think about some of the negative things that have happened to you: bullying, teasing, shaming, or lies spoken over you in a moment of unrestrained rage or overwhelming fear. Now stop and think about how the negative energy that was spewed on you had been carried inside someone who was passing on the pain dumped onto them. Before they hurt you, someone had hurt them, and before that, someone had hurt that person too. All that painful emotional energy flows on and on.

I like to think of generational sin as an echo of the first law of thermodynamics. For instance, my client Sandy came from a home in which both of her parents were so obese that they needed regular medical care and took a daily menu of medications. From a very young age, Sandy was told that she was destined to face the same battle with her weight and she should get used to the fact that this was in their family genes. Sandy's future looked bleak, so food became an even closer comfort and friend, especially on the days she was bullied, teased, and called fat.

By the time Sandy got to college, her five-foot-three frame was eighty pounds overweight and in need of daily insulin. Winded every time she had to climb a flight of stairs at Pepperdine University (a hillside university known for its beautiful ocean views), Sandy took matters into her own hands freshman year. She turned to extreme dieting and exercise. A diet soda and a pack of gum a day were her daily indulgences—delicacies. She dropped the eighty pounds and then some, but all the extreme working out and dieting caused her body distress, showing up in hair loss, eczema, anemia, and sky-high cholesterol.

When Sandy came to see me, she was in post-graduate school. By then, the extra weight had returned along with an extra fifteen pounds. Sandy had grown up loving Jesus and knew something had to change. But now she recognized that she couldn't solely focus on her caloric energy. She started meeting with me along with a trauma specialist. Instead of focusing on diet culture and extreme fitness, we began the slow and steady process of helping Sandy get back in her body while letting God kindly love and lead her, as you will do through this book's Metabolize sections. She learned to live in her body and tend to her emotional energy with a foundation of loving-kindness. As her heart became more like Christ's, Sandy was able to see that the lies she had believed were not her parents' fault; the same handbook of lies had been passed down to them from their own parents.

When there is no one to teach children how to process their negative emotional energy and show them how to metabolize pain into goodness, compassion, and empathy, lies are easily passed down the family line. If that was your experience, I have good news: God is the creator, initiator, and sustainer of all good things, including His Word. Remember the first law of thermodynamics? Likewise, God's Word can't be created or destroyed, but it can take bad things and change them into something that brings goodness. If we apply God's Word to our lives when bad things happen to us, we have power to change our thinking, feeling, and choosing from negativity into goodness.

God is transforming all things back to the state of being good. Using heat, I was able to change my beaker of ice in chemistry class into water that then bubbled up into steam. Likewise, in Christ, we can be transformed into a new state of being—from merely surviving to thriving. Instead of hating what we see in the mirror, we can begin to celebrate and bless what we see. We can move from counting calories to counting our blessings; from weighing our bodies to weighing our hearts. In Christ, we can become completely new.

In Christ, we can be transformed into a new state
of being—from merely surviving to thriving.

We are transformed into people who reflect God's glory when God's Word has renewed our minds and given us new hearts that desire what God wants, ears to hear what God is saying, and empowering grace to do what God is doing. Our bodies then become the instrument for administering God's will to a world in need. If we want to know who we are, it begins with knowing who He is.

Make it a point to train your body to fill your negative space (your energy) with more of Him. You will never be the same. Filling your mind with the thoughts and ideas of heaven is just what your soul craves.

The love of God changes everything. There's nothing His love can't transform. His love melts our frozen hearts so we can take in His living water and then challenges us to believe that there is more power available to us than we can see.

Energy can't be created or destroyed. All energy is used. Raise your hand if you want your energy to be used well!

The Metabolism of the Holy Spirit

My two children did more to forge my heart during their adolescence than at any other time. If you have a teenager or have raised one, you know those years aren't the easiest. These young adults without fully formed brains are learning, growing, and stretching out into the world as they become their own persons—the persons God created them to be. We parents get to learn, grow, and stretch more into who we were created to be whenever they bring us pain to be metabolized with God.

Parenting is a gift, a pleasure, but that doesn't mean it always *feels* pleasant. Through my children, I have learned more about the sin that Jesus wants to love out of me. Fear and control are often the first to rise up. When my children tell me the hard truth about what they're facing or a poor choice they've made, I just want to fix it, save them, and keep them away from the bad things that go bump in the night. But I can't. I can't be their God.

One morning I woke with an ache in my chest after a long night of tossing and turning while worrying about my kids. Fear had been having a rager of a slumber party in my bed all night. I woke up, took a deep breath, and exhaled, "Jesus, help." Then these words rose in my spirit: *Alisa, don't you know it's the job of My Holy Spirit to help you eat adversity for breakfast and poop joy by lunch?* Cleary, I had been studying the body's metabolism and thermodynamics that week. The Lord was speaking to me in the language in which I was seeking Him.

Remember, metabolism is the process of sustaining life, which requires something to go in so something can come out. Food fuels us for needed energy, and extra energy comes out as waste. I propose that it's the Holy Spirit's job to take the "wood" of what we think and feel, and run it through the furnace of Truth. This keeps us from doing or saying something that perpetuates pain and leaves a stain on our soul or someone else's. Instead of producing waste, the Holy Spirit helps us process our pain until out comes joy! In my case, the Spirit reminded me that He loves my kids even more than I do and was at work in their current circumstances.

> When the Spirit of truth comes, he will guide you into all the truth, for he will not speak on his own authority, but whatever he hears he will speak, and he will declare to you the things that are to come.
> JOHN 6:13
>
> I have told you this so that my joy may be in you and that your joy may be complete.
> JOHN 15:11, NIV

Satan, the enemy of our transformation, is openly put to shame every time a follower of Christ chooses to exchange a lie for God's truth. He definitely hates it whenever the children of God experience joy rather than pain!

When I read Luke 4, when Jesus rolled open the scroll of Isaiah and delivered His first sermon in his local synagogue, I imagine a connection between His words and the first law of thermodynamics. In other words, God turns to good all that the world considers waste:

The Spirit of the LORD is on me,
  because he has anointed me
  to proclaim good news to the poor.
He has sent me to proclaim freedom for the prisoners
  and recovery of sight for the blind,
  to set the oppressed free,
to proclaim the year of the LORD's favor.

Then he rolled up the scroll, gave it back to the attendant and sat down. The eyes of everyone in the synagogue were fastened on him. He began by saying to them, "Today this scripture is fulfilled in your hearing."
LUKE 4:18-21

So let's get this straight:

The people who feel bankrupt receive Good News.
The prisoners who feel stuck receive liberty.
The blind gain sight.
Anyone bound (mentally, emotionally, or physically) becomes free.

With God nothing is wasted. This is all good news—and not just good news for our souls but for our bodies too! Jesus was declaring that a higher reality of heaven had arrived! In this reality, nothing remains stuck, and everyone has access to God's transforming love. The Son of God put on skin and made the unseen seen to break us free from all our chains of pain. Jesus didn't come to show us Himself in the flesh just so we would believe; He came to show us the way to *be* in our bodies as we believe. Jesus knew how to take everything coming against Him and turn it into something that could bring more good news. And now, because of God's Holy Spirit in us, we have a greater strength for the ability to think, feel, and choose as God would have us to.

Like Jesus, we can learn to contain this Good News in our bodies and give it away too!

——— Metabolize ———

Mind

1. How does knowing that energy can't be created or destroyed but only transformed or transmitted change the way you think about your body's health?
2. When it comes to your health, what would it look like for the Holy Spirit to take the pain of your adversity and turn it into joy?

Mouth

Father God, come deliver me from anything that has come against me to try and chain me to my pain. Take me out of this frozen state of being and turn me into the Holy Spirit's steam. Amen.

Move

Use this link for your kind-mind renewing movement that goes along with this chapter: https://www.revelationwellness.org/tbr/move/.

CHAPTER 4

GOD'S BURNING DESIRE FOR YOU

JENNIFER SNUCK INTO MY FITNESS class every week. Well-connected in the local community, she was known for bringing light and laughter into any room and for throwing good parties. Having Jennifer in class was like having the most popular girl in high school sit at your table in the cafeteria. Initially, Jennifer wasn't too sure about Jesus and His words, which I sometimes talked about during class, but something brought her back each week. Although she probably told her friends she came for the convenient calorie burn, I suspected the real reason was her interest in knowing more about God.

Jennifer ran regularly and had the sleek, lean physical build of an Olympic runner. Running in at least three marathons a year, she placed in the top ten of her age group every time. She'd been running since high school and loved the natural high she felt when her feet kicked up dust for miles on end. Although she was very athletic, I noticed something interesting about Jennifer. Whenever she walked across the room, it was very robotically. Her head seemed to float over her rounded shoulders while the rest of her body moved swift and rigidly. The language of her body communicated anxious and guarded energy. Over time she asked me questions about God and confided in me about her hidden struggle with her body image. One day, as we talked over a cup of coffee, she took her right hand, grabbed her right thigh until it left a mark on her skin, and told me with disgust, "It doesn't matter how much I run, or how little I eat, all I see is fat. Fat, fat, fat! I can't stand what I see."

The more I got to know Jennifer, the better I understood why she felt such disdain for her body and seemed disconnected from it. Jennifer had endured a very challenging childhood. When she was only five years old, her mother left her father, her, and her younger brother, who had intellectual disabilities. Her father quickly remarried a woman who was jealous of Jennifer and resented having to care for her brother. Her stepmother was verbally unkind and sometimes physically cruel. As a result, Jennifer felt it was up to her to mother her brother while also caring for her father by never revealing how unkind her stepmother could be. Jennifer was good at keeping the peace. She kept trouble neatly tucked away by learning to wear a variety of masks that enabled her to be whomever the current situation needed her to be. Because she always suppressed her own needs, the hidden pain inside her continued to build. After a high school track teacher mentioned that he saw the extra weight she'd put on over summer break of her sophomore year, she developed an eating disorder. Eventually her emotional suppression resulted in dangerous drinking, drugs, and sexual encounters in college. Each encounter felt good in the moment but came with a backlash of shame.

Now Jennifer was showing up weekly to my class, looking for a safe place to be herself and longing for tranquility. She was finding peace as she moved her body in the presence of God and other people who felt kind and safe. Sometimes after a workout, she would tell me about how she'd just encountered the presence of God's peace in her body, something she had never felt before. God's love was pursuing Jennifer.

But after a few months of growing closer to Jesus, Jennifer turned back and metaphorically ran away. She told me that issues were starting to reemerge that were too scary for her to deal with, even bringing up some old thoughts and tendencies that brought more feelings of shame. She was having a hard time reconciling a God who loves her with a God who allowed her to go through so much pain—and now seemed to be bringing it back up. In His love, the Holy Spirit was starting to bring to Jennifer's mind some of the pain in her past. God's Word, which is a lamp, was illuminating some of the dark places in Jennifer's heart but it was freaking her out. She stopped coming to class and returned to running, but she did start going to therapy.

You may wonder why God allowed Jennifer to experience such fear, knowing it would only cause her to run from Him. Because God is perfect love and light, He wants us to know that, with Him, we don't have to be afraid of the dark. Little by little, in the illumination of God's love, the shameful and painful places of our past will be exposed to the light and healed—as long as we don't run away. Fear that causes us to run from God is not from God. We mustn't be afraid of the dark.

From the Beginning

Have you ever wondered why God, "in the beginning" (Genesis 1:1), created everything knowing it would all go south? He knew we would listen to an enemy who only wants to kill, steal, and destroy, thus disobeying our Creator and allowing sin to enter the world. I mean, what gives, God? Why all the beauty and why all the pain?

One day, my son, Jack, asked me a similar question as I was driving him to school. "Mama, why would God create us knowing we were going to mess it all up?"

As I glanced back in the rearview mirror, I said, "Because no matter what, God wanted kids. It's just like how your dad and I wanted you and your sister, knowing that it wouldn't be easy, that we wouldn't be perfect parents, and that you two wouldn't be perfect children. We still wanted a family. We wanted kids."

And with those words, Jack got it. Unconditional love isn't reasonable. Unconditional love doesn't always feel good, and it doesn't always make sense. In the beginning, God—fully content as Father, Son, and Holy Spirit—still desired a bigger family. God wanted kids! He knew His children would go through troubles, but He also knew those troubles would help to make them more like His Son, Jesus, who was sent to make a way for us to get back to our Father's home.

As you continue through the warm-up phase and then move into the more intense part of the workout for metabolizing your pain, please remember this as the reason for continuing: You were created to desire God because He first desired you. God will not stop desiring you!

We love because God first loved us. In fact, God's desire for you is stronger than your desire for a better body, outlasts your craving for something sweet to eat, and outpaces your attempts to run away from Him.

Long before God designed all that we can see, He had us in mind. He created a perfect place where His children could grow, learn, and explore. Then God made males and females, the only beings created in His image. He placed them in the center of His creation, hoping they would choose to walk, talk, think, and do life like Him: "Long before he laid down earth's foundations, he had us in mind, had settled on us as the focus of his love, to be made whole and holy by his love" (Ephesians 1:4, MSG). The reason you desire anything good is because the God who defines good first desired you. He put flesh and bones around you, and He called you good. You are God's good idea! Don't let the bad things that have happened rip you off from the good that God has for you!

Contrary to what the world says, it's a waste of time and energy to work only for a shapely body that you love to show off, but it's never a waste of time to desire a body that thinks, feels, and chooses to express God's love. Because God first loved us, being kind to our bodies is an act of multiplying love.

Knowing that you were first loved by God and always desired by Him will give you the staying power to allow your pain to be transformed into purpose when the less than comfortable things show up. Christ's love can keep you from turning and running the other way as Jennifer did. For goodness' sake, don't quit! Remember that you have an enemy whose desire is to ruin you by keeping you from God: "Be sober-minded; be watchful. Your adversary the devil prowls around like a roaring lion, seeking someone to devour" (1 Peter 5:8).

An Eternal, Enduring Love

Earlier we introduced the parable of the Prodigal Son, found in Luke 15. Jesus began to tell this story to a crowd of tax collectors, sinners, and religious leaders: "There was a man who had two sons" (verse 11).

And with that opening sentence, Jesus cut to the heart of everyone with ears to hear. They perked up because everyone listening had a family—from the tax collector with money hidden under his bed but no peace to the religious leader with lots of followers but no love. Despite their differences, all of them had some experience of home and family.

Like Jennifer, some people have experienced a lot of family pain; others have an upbringing that spared them a lot of heartache. But I would venture a guess and say that you are reading this book because, though you love God, His love feels far away right now. You don't embody His love, but you would like to. And I propose this is why: It's hard to love and feel close to the God who made you when you don't love the body you have, the one you see when you look in the mirror. When you dislike your body, the love you experience from God and the love you feel toward Him will feel fractured and distant.

It's like when a friend gives you a tacky gift that you feel obligated to display. The relationship begins to feel a bit strained and awkward. You don't stop loving your friend, but when gift-giving time comes again, you hold your breath. When it comes to your body, you can stop holding your breath. Instead, be thankful for this amazing gift, which supports one of the greatest gifts you've been given—*life!*

Here's good news: God, the Father, who oversees creation, loves *all* His kids. He desires to make you "whole and holy by His love" Ephesians 1:4 (MSG), to teach you howto remain in His love. Because of Jesus, God's love has now moved into your body, your home here on earth. In this home, God's love chases out all your fear. This is important because, while fear can get the wheels of change turning, only the love of God can sustain real and lasting change.

God desires to make you "whole and holy by His love."

God, your Father in heaven, desired you since eternity past. He has no plans of giving up on you. His love will never stop pursuing you and transforming you from the inside out. All you need do is to stop running and blaming.

Whether you seek physical, emotional, or mental change, if you want to be in sync with the most significant transforming force in the world, get in step with God's desires. Get to know His heart and what He burns for, and things are sure to happen.

God's love is an eternal fire of desire that burns for His children on earth. When He reveals His goodness through you, God's glory is seen. His love is not a dumpster fire that trashes people but a consuming fire that transforms people. Or as the Bible explains, God's fire results in sanctification—the process through which life's difficulties are used for good as they expose your weaknesses and need for God. His fierce and fiery love shows up and burns away the junk inside you. Troubles in this world expose the sin that sneakily entangles and weighs you down. No wonder James was inspired by the Holy Spirit to write these words of encouragement:

> Count it all joy, my brothers, when you meet trials of various kinds, for you know that the testing of your faith produces steadfastness. And let steadfastness have its full effect, that you may be perfect and complete, lacking in nothing.
>
> JAMES 1:2-4, ESV

God's love is not a dumpster fire that trashes people but a consuming fire that transforms people.

Remaining in God's love is an endurance event. And all endurance athletes need sustained hydration. Through His Word, Christ offers us living water that is far more refreshing, sustaining, and energizing than the hydration we think we'll get by gaining others' approval or garnering more likes on social media.

Just as surely as the sun will rise and set each day, what God desires to accomplish through all your ups and downs will be done. Stay close to God's love, His energy. His love has the power to transform you, setting and keeping you free.

Metabolize

Mind

1. What thoughts or feelings come to mind when you hear the phrase "God desires you"?
2. List all the emotions you feel when you desire things that make you feel good in the moment but don't offer lasting benefits.
3. God wants to transform your life's disappointments into the fuel for your divine destiny. How does thinking this way about your struggles change your view of pain?
4. What Bible passage in this chapter spoke to you most? Write it down and explain what God is specifically saying to you through that verse.

Mouth

God, I need You to move into my body and make Yourself at home. Show me the things I need to know about how my heart was meant to feel and how my mind was designed to think. I want only to transform and transmit joy, not pain. I've been afraid to let You move in completely because of the lies I've believed about love. Shine Your healing love and light into me and keep me from running away in fear. Show me and teach me Your ways to supreme love. Amen.

Move

Be sure to water your body and brain. Water makes up 60 percent of your body and 73 percent of your heart and brain.[1] Water is to our body-brain connection what motor oil is to our cars. Without oil in a car, the engine is at risk of going up in flames. And so it is for us when we don't have a well-watered body and brain. If you struggle with low energy, brain fog, body aches, and headaches, be sure to pay attention to your body's engine warning light and ask yourself this important question: *Am I getting enough water?*

Make it your goal to drink half your body weight in ounces of water each day. For example, if you weigh 140 pounds, you should drink at least 70 ounces of water daily.

Also, today and going forward, we are going to add another practice for processing our pain at the end of each chapter. I invite you to practice a quick, ten-minute biblical mind-body meditation—a time for you to be still and be loved. Perhaps the thought of sitting still makes you anxious. Just know, if that's true for you, a powerful and effective tool for healing your body and brain connection awaits you. Research confirms the benefits of meditation, especially for those who want to improve their physical, mental, and emotional health. You will learn more about the benefits of meditation in an upcoming chapter, but I don't want you to have to wait to start reaping the benefits.

Use this link for your Be Still and Be Loved meditation that goes along with this chapter: https://www.revelationwellness.org/tbr/still/. I encourage you, as I always encourage my clients, to use your journal to record any visuals or words that come to mind after your time of stillness or movement.

Use this link to access this chapter's kind-mind renewing movement: https://www.revelationwellness.org/tbr/move/.

Recognizing Our Pain

*Not many days later, the younger son gathered all he
had and took a journey into a far country, and there he
squandered his property in reckless living. And when he had
spent everything, a severe famine arose in that country.*

LUKE 15:13-14

CHAPTER 5

PAIN AND THE EARLY BODY AND BRAIN

I WAS FOURTEEN WHEN MY MOM CALLED my brother and me into my brother's bedroom. Her steps were heavy as we followed her. As she closed the door, she told us to sit down because she had something to tell us. *What now?* I thought. *Did I leave my room a mess again? Did I leave my shoes on the floor in the den? What did I do wrong this time?* As my brother and I huddled next to each other on his twin bed, my heart moved into my throat and I braced for impact.

"I think you both should know that your father has been unfaithful to me," my mom said in a stern but steady voice. "And last month, he was picked up by the police for soliciting a prostitute. He's been arrested and convicted for solicitation and will be serving time in jail on the weekends for the next few months."

Suddenly, I thought of all the times my father had told us he was running out to get us ice cream and never came back home. Now it made sense. My father desired other women just like his own father had. His inheritance of misplaced desire had now landed with the impact of a bomb exploding, hitting our little family of four with the fallout of pain.

I suppose my mom hoped that by telling us the extent of our father's betrayal, he would be shamed into changing. But like fear, while shame might motivate a person to change, it has no power to sustain the momentum. Although I am sure my mom felt a little lighter after unloading our family secret on her two young teens, I certainly didn't feel better—just angrier and inflamed. Mom had passed her pain on to me.

This was the moment everything shifted in the way I saw the world and other people—and not in a good way. A flame of rebellious anger had been lit inside me, and I used this angry energy to find the quickest way out of my parents' house. Like the Prodigal Son in Luke 15:12-13, I started making plans to gather all I had to journey into a far-off country. But in my case, I wanted to get far, far away from the house of pain where I'd spent my childhood.

Little did I know that my unprocessed pain would follow me into adulthood and negatively affect both my body and my brain.

The ACE Study

In the 1980s, researchers at Kaiser Permanente in San Diego studied clinically obese patients. Dr. Vincent Felitti had created an extraordinarily successful weight-loss program in which participants would successfully and safely lose up to three hundred pounds in one year. But after five years of administering this program, Dr. Felitti and his team discovered a big problem: 50 percent of people who were successfully losing weight dropped out. This attrition frustrated him, so he began to probe deeper to determine why. When he interviewed people who'd left the program, he found that a majority had experienced childhood sexual abuse. Felitti knew he was on to something more significant than the need to help people manage their weight; they were also dealing with lingering internal mental health issues like depression, anxiety, and fear due to trauma.

Between 1995 and 1997, Felitti joined forces with Dr. Robert Anda and the Centers for Disease Control to create the Adverse Childhood Experiences Study. After 13,000 people went through a thorough medical evaluation to detail their current health condition, including physical discomforts and diagnoses, they were sent a questionnaire with just ten queries about their childhood. Five of the questions asked whether they had experienced one or more of the following: sexual abuse, physical abuse, emotional abuse, physical neglect, or emotional neglect. The other five were specific to the adverse environments in which they were raised, asking if they had grown up in a home directly impacted by divorce, separation, or death; mental illness, domestic violence; substance abuse; or incarceration. For each question they answered yes, they were given one point toward their overall ACE score.[1]

The results were shocking.

Of the 13,000 people, 70 percent responded to the survey. Over half of them answered yes to one or more of the questions, meaning they had experienced some form of childhood adversity before the age of eighteen.

In her book *Childhood Disrupted*, author Donna Jackson Nakazawa explains the correlation between our exposure to childhood adversity and its effects on our physical health as grown adults:

> How many categories of Adverse Childhood Experiences patients had encountered could by and large predict how much medical care they would require in adulthood: the higher one's ACE Score, the higher the number of doctor visits they'd had in the past year, and the higher their number of unexplained physical symptoms.
>
> People with an ACE Score of 4 were twice as likely to be diagnosed with cancer than someone with an ACE Score of 0. For each ACE Score an individual had, the chance of being hospitalized with an autoimmune disease in adulthood rose to 20 percent. Someone with an ACE Score of 4 was 460 percent more likely to be facing depression than someone with a score of 0.
>
> An ACE Score of 6 and higher shortened an individual's lifespan by almost twenty years.[2]

According to Harvard University's Center on the Developing Child, excessive and ongoing childhood stress disrupts the structure and development of a child's brain: "When children experience toxic stress, their cortisol levels remain elevated for prolonged periods of time. Both animal and human studies show that long-term elevations in cortisol levels can alter the function of a number of neural systems, suppress the immune response, and even change the architecture of regions in the brain that are essential for learning and memory."[3]

A disrupted brain structure will make it feel darn near impossible for a person to think, say, and do the right thing, especially in moments when the key motivation is simply to survive and get through them. It's no wonder that people who are stressed reach for comfort foods, which are usually comprised primarily of sugars and starches.

When our minds perceive a threat, the stress hormone cortisol is released by the adrenal glands. Cortisol increases sugars (glucose) in the bloodstream, making quick energy available for the working muscles in our body so they can fight or flee, getting us out of danger and to safety. If we are in a dangerous situation, like being chased by a bear, cortisol is a godsend. But if "the bear" lives in our home, comes home drunk every night, isn't available to meet our needs, and threatens our safety, our stress levels may stay chronically high.

When stressed, the immune system becomes disturbed and the body can experience inflammation, which is its proactive response to threat (more on inflammation to come). But if adversity has reorganized our brains so we live with ongoing stress because we fear "the bear," chronic inflammation occurs. Sustained inflammation negatively affects our immune system, making us more prone to physical sickness and disease.[4] In fact, researchers report that stress plays a role in up to 90 percent of all sickness and disease.[5]

If you grew up in difficult circumstances and are feeling triggered or hopeless by the description of ACEs, now is the time to take hope in Jesus—a living hope. Scripture tells us that Jesus' posture toward us is one of love and compassion. Consider His response when He saw the crowds who had followed Him during His time on earth: "He had compassion for them, because they were harassed and helpless, like sheep without a shepherd" (Matthew 9:36). Remember this as you follow God's design for moving through the pain of your past:

1. We must not stress (aka worry).
2. We must learn how to process pain in proper and healthy ways.

In His famous Sermon on the Mount, Jesus introduces people to God's Kingdom, which is unlike anything the people had heard of. He says, "I tell you, do not be anxious about your life, what you will eat or what you will drink, nor about your body, what you will put on" (Matthew 6:25). While that might have been a novel instruction to them, it permeates Scripture: I've heard that the Bible says, "Do not fear" at least 365 times, one verse for each day of the year. Yes, God means it when He says we are not to fear (be anxious, worried, or stressed). It's not that fear is impolite and unbecoming of His children; rather, I believe He tells us not to fear because living stressed, anxious, afraid, or worried rips at the very thread of our design. Ongoing stress destroys our health, overwhelms our nervous system, disrupts the body-brain connection, and makes it hard for God's perfect peace and presence to remain within us. The first step to healing is to stop living in fear and stress.

Second, we must learn to properly process our pain. When Jesus talked about His Kingdom, He didn't pull any punches. He tells only the truth, which is why He said that in this world we would have trouble. Then He added that we are to take heart because He has overcome everything that attempts to overcome us (John 16:33).

We must learn to take heart! We do so when we endure pain without hurting ourselves or others. We can learn to feel pain without letting it overtake us. We take heart when we remember who we are, who we belong to, and the Kingdom from which we have been sent. (We'll dive deeper into all of this when we move into the workout and cooldown phases.)

We take heart when we remember who we are, who we belong to, and the Kingdom from which we have been sent.

When I was younger, I hadn't learned how to take heart and process my pain. As a result, I became "an expresser"—someone who was easily inflamed and overreacted to innocent offenses.

Other people repress their pain. These people often come from fairly "tidy" homes where emotions were scarcely seen and barely heard. They may have an ACE score of one or zero but feel emotionally flat and unattached. These "repressors" feel it is unsafe to express what they feel, want, or need. In order to conform to someone else's needs, repressors bury desire or, to put it another way, they let their pain hibernate. Yet when this sleeping giant awakens, it finds its way out of the body in the form of physical symptoms like headaches and stomach pain. As Gabor Maté writes in *When the Body Says No*, "When we have been prevented from learning how to say no our bodies may end up saying it for us."[6] If your ACE score is zero and none of these scenarios resonate with you but you are familiar with life's pain, please keep reading. There's a reason you picked up this book.

Our inability to become the people we so desperately want to be—men and women who reflect what God's Word tells us we can be—is due not only to our lack of self-control or knowledge of Scripture. Being raised in unsafe, unpredictable, and unattached environments may have rewired our brains to do what was necessary to survive adversity and stay safe.

If you rarely or inconsistently felt safe and loved growing up—if you didn't know whether you would be hugged or hurt, cheered or jeered from one day to the next—your body and brain have probably been running scared. The ever-present high levels of cortisol in your nervous system keep you living on high alert. Couple this inherited stress with the fast-paced, smartphone, technology-based world, and it's no wonder you struggle to make and sustain change.

Trying to love God and others with a brain trained and neurologically ingrained to run on stress and fear can be overwhelming. It can make us feel insane, like we are doing the same things repeatedly and hoping for new results. As Christians, going to church, reading our Bibles, singing worship songs, and checking all the spiritual boxes of activity can keep us busy while failing to deliver a fulfilling, joyful life. Jesus offers a better way. He said He came not to help us survive but to *thrive*:

> A thief is only there to steal and kill and destroy. I came so they can have real and eternal life, more and better life than they ever dreamed of.
>
> JOHN 10:10, MSG

Without a deep awareness that we are loved, chosen, wanted, covered, and fought for by God, our minds will stay stuck in survival mode and our bodies will be more susceptible to sickness and dis-ease. Head knowledge alone won't solve the problem. We need an embodied knowledge of God's love for us, the ability to sense His presence and peace. That is what the Metabolize section at the end of each chapter is designed to do. Without the renewed mind of God and embodied knowledge gained through our minds, mouths, and movement, even the most devout believer will have difficulty experiencing complete transformation.

> *We need an embodied knowledge of God's love for us,*
> *the ability to sense His presence and peace.*

It doesn't matter how many push-ups and squats we do, miles we run, salads we eat, or Bible studies we attend. If we don't process how our past has stressed our bodies, negatively affects our brains, influences the way we view the present, and interferes with our ability to have hope for the future, we don't stand a chance of living a healthy and whole life. A vibrant life of joy comes from God and is our strength.

If you grew up experiencing adversity or if now, as an adult, you live in a constant state of stress and physical pain, I wish I could place my hands on your shoulders and square you up to look me in the eyes. I would then tell you clearly and with authority: "It's not your fault." Your inability to make positive and sustainable health change is not your fault. The reason you struggle with your health isn't because there's something wrong with you.

As I've worked with thousands of people who feel dissatisfied with their bodies, I've discovered that their inability to make good choices is often due to never learning what to do with the wrong (the sin) that's been done to them. As a result, they continue to feed the cycle of pain by thinking and choosing wrong.

"The first step to healing," wrote Henri Nouwen, "is not a step away from the pain but a step toward it."[7] For that reason, I urge you to keep practicing the Metabolize portions of this book to help you rewire your brain-body circuitry. The Spirit of God—the One who lives inside you and knows what's best for your body and brain—*is* your personal trainer. The Holy Spirit, partnered with the active, alive Word of God, has the power to re-architect and organize your brain, renew your mind, and restore your connection to your body in a way that is loving and kind.

How's that for good news?

Metabolize

Mind

The questions to the ACE study appear on pages 272–273. In the spirit of learning to metabolize pain, I encourage you to ask yourself those ten questions. Please note: If you aren't sure whether a question is true for you, but it has felt true, consider that a subtle yes. Give yourself one point for each question to which you respond yes.

Please note: Many of these questions could be triggering if you had a difficult childhood. Pray and ask the Holy Spirit to guide you and comfort you as you answer them. Or if you don't think it would be a good idea to answer these questions without the presence of a trained counselor, feel free to push on and keep reading.

And just so you know that we are in this together, my ACE score is a 6.

Mouth

Say the following prayer aloud. Repeat it a few times if that's what it takes to believe it.

Father God, thank You that You did not leave me as an orphan. You've adopted me into Your family and given me a new home. In this place, I can rest. In Your love, I can trust. Holy Spirit, I give You access to the structure and organization of my brain. Begin Your work of healing my mind until my body lives in good health and my soul prospers. Amen.

Move

Use this link for your kind-mind renewing movement: https://www.revelation wellness.org/tbr/move/.

Follow this link for the Be Still and Be Loved meditation that goes along with this chapter: https://www.revelationwellness.org/tbr/still/.

CHAPTER 6

HOW PAIN CHANGES YOUR BODY AND BRAIN

CONNIE SHOWS UP FOR OUR 7 A.M. training session a little late. She had another restless night, tossing and turning in her sheets. Connie is forty-two and married to a kind man who loves the Lord. He thinks Connie is beautiful. He tells her he loves her no matter her size or weight. But Connie has a hard time believing him. Though she loves her husband, she struggles with feeling safe and attached to him. Since giving birth to her three children, now teens, she's experienced a host of ailments. Her body no longer feels like her own. Year after year, her body continues to host unruly and uninvited visitors like migraine headaches, gastrointestinal issues, and phantom body aches, which sometimes make it hard for her to get out of bed and move. She attributes her health problems to the weight she's put on over the years.

One day while walking and running intervals, Connie confides in me something that embarrasses her even more than the size of her stomach—her emotional outbursts over small matters. Connie is a good mom and a loving wife and friend, but she worries about bad things happening to the people she loves. And to make matters worse, because Connie loves Jesus, the shame she feels after "losing it" with others, especially her children, leaves her feeling even more ashamed, afraid, and disgusted with herself. So Connie turns to food to comfort herself when she feels bad. That's because food never talks back or lets her down like some of the people she loves. As we walk side by side, she says, "I swear some days I feel like I am crazy! I read God's Word and try to do what it says, but something's wrong. Alisa, what's wrong with my brain?"

"Actually," I say, "there's nothing wrong with you. Your brain is doing exactly what it is was made to do."

Noting her surprised look, I take a few minutes to briefly explain the difference between our brains and our minds. To provide us with more context for this chapter, I'll go a bit deeper than I did with Connie. The brain is made of spongy soft tissue, coiled around in stacked tubes, safely tucked beneath layers of protective tissue and fluid—all of which are inside twenty-two bones that form a protective helmet-like structure. It's filled with approximately 86 billion neurons (cells that transmit impulses), which communicate in trillions of connections called synapses. Our brains have both chemical and electrical synapses, making it possible for us to use our minds to express ourselves through infinite thoughts, emotions, desires, and will. It keeps our bodies' systems functioning without our conscious thought.

But when it comes to making deliberate choices and movement, the brain waits for us to tell it what to do. I like to compare the brain to a personal butler who shows up to serve you. You give an order with a thought in your mind, and the brain responds, "As you wish!" For example, if you notice that a coworker isn't being kind to you, your brain looks for input and information to back up that thought. (*She didn't even say hello when I passed her in the hall. . . . I heard her joking with the receptionist, so she must just be mad at me. . . . I bet she doesn't like the changes I made to her draft of the report.*) The brain is accommodating and will give you more of what you ask for as you think.

While your brain waits to receive information from you, your mind is where the real, one-of-a-kind you made in God's image resides. It is the seat of your consciousness, your awareness. It draws from your memories and experiences to form your ideas, biases, personal preferences, worldview, and beliefs about yourself in relation to the world around you. You make meaning of the world through your mind, which shapes your understanding of the way life works.

Now let's consider another simple analogy that shows how the brain, mind, and body all work together. Your brain is like your car's engine—a hunk of metal with a battery, gears, pistons, and other assorted parts. With a full tank of gas (thanks to food and water), your engine (brain) is a revved-up motor ready to go wherever you want. But without a driver, the car (your body) can't go anywhere. Your mind is the driver. Your mind sits in the driver's seat and takes the vehicle of your body wherever you want to go. Hopefully, it's in the direction that God is moving.

Proverbs 23:7 says, "As [someone] thinks within himself, so he is." As someone thinks, so she is, sitting behind the wheel of her mind, deciding where she wants to go. In Connie's case, if she thinks she is ugly and fat and is disgusted with her body, so she will be. Over the years, her brain had continually fired synapses, forming neuropathways. Think of neuropathways as the routes our thoughts take. When we think a specific thought repeatedly through the years, we turn a remote single-track trail in the wilderness of our mind into an easy-to-access highway. These paths of thought Connie had traveled told her that she wasn't enough and that the world was a dangerous place. Her brain then wired all these messages together. They had become strong thoughts traveling in her brain, but she had learned she could find momentary relief in brownies or potato chips. The more she traveled these paths in her "car," the more she strengthened and confirmed her negative outlook on life and eventually found her car in the body shop known as her pantry.

"Neurons that fire together wire together" helps explain this automatic phenomenon. Although our brain is gracious in confirming our biases and giving us more of what we want, it's also lazy. The brain looks for the path of least resistance so it can conserve energy, the energy we need to survive. If the way we dealt with a stressful moment in the past helped us survive the moment and kept us safe, we are most likely to do the same thing in the future. Because the network of thought gets stronger and stronger with use, we continue to travel those familiar pathways. And we wonder why, after getting a phone call that brings bad news, we find ourselves halfway through a package of cookies or a gallon of ice cream. When trouble comes, our brain's instinct is to do what it's always done to serve us and keep us safe. We must teach our brain that there's a better way—the way of a renewed mind.

The brain looks for the path of least resistance
so it can conserve energy and survive.

Because we were created in God's image, our life works best when we think, feel, and choose like He does. When we don't, the way our bodies and brains work can be negatively affected. To help make sense of this breakdown in our design, think about what happens when a person accidentally puts diesel fuel into a car. The car won't go far before it backfires, stammers, and eventually stalls.

As the apostle Paul begins to sign off his letter to the church at Philippi, he writes,

> Finally, brothers, whatever is true, whatever is honorable,
> whatever is just, whatever is pure, whatever is lovely, whatever
> is commendable, if there is any excellence, if there is anything
> worthy of praise, *think* about these things.
> PHILIPPIANS 4:8, EMPHASIS MINE

In this verse, Paul tells you the kind of fuel your body needs for life to go as God intended! Fill your mind with thoughts of God and His goodness so you can get in your body and use your brain to do the good work you've been created to do.

Our brains can help us survive and stay alive, but when our minds are renewed by God's Word, they can work with our bodies to do good deeds, giving us the ability to transform pain on this earth into the purposes of heaven. If what we think doesn't line up with God's perspective, we can notice the "check engine" light, quickly pull over, and bring the car to a stop. Idling roadside, we can take a moment to breathe, reset, and renew our minds with what God has said. We can then get back on the road and go in a different direction at a slower, more gentle pace.

As we learned in chapter 5, the adversity we experience, especially early in life, affects our brain's structure and organization, making it difficult for us to think, feel, and choose the right road in troubling moments. So we can create a better map to guide us when trouble comes, let's take a moment to define and classify this pain.

Trauma: The Unwelcome Resident in Our Brains

In a word, adverse circumstances can lead to trauma, which the Substance Abuse and Mental Health Services Administration says results "from an event, series of events, or set of circumstances that is experienced by an individual as physically or emotionally harmful or life threatening and that has lasting adverse effects on the individual's functioning and mental, physical, social, emotional, or spiritual well-being."[1]

Notice how multifaceted trauma can be. It can affect our minds and bodies, as well as our relationships with others and with God. It's also good to note that trauma is rooted in someone's experience. Two people can go through the same challenging moment and come out with two very different experiences. If someone believes an event was traumatic for them, we should believe them. It's their experience, not ours.

There are two categories, or types, of trauma; big *T* and little *t*. Big *T* traumas are extraordinary situations in which a person's life or body is threatened. They stem from living through natural disasters, catastrophic car accidents, physical and sexual abuse, or violent crimes, or from witnessing or participating in war. These traumas are a violation of our bodies, where they are felt deeply. Helplessness is a key factor of big *T* traumas. When people are held against their will, violently attacked, or deprived of resources needed for survival, they will most likely neither fight nor take flight but freeze.

Small *t* traumas stretch us beyond our ability to cope, causing emotional distress. These are not life- or body-threatening events but violations against our self-importance—what we would want or do. Some examples of little *t* traumas are relational conflict; infidelity; being bullied, shamed, or teased; emotional abuse; legal trouble; financial worries; and the loss of a pet or significant loved one. Often we try to minimize their effects on us:

> Small 't' traumas tend to be overlooked by the individual who has experienced the difficulty. This is sometimes due to the tendency to rationalize the experience as common and therefore cognitively shame oneself for any reaction that could be construed as an over-reaction or being "dramatic."[2]

There's no debate that big *T* traumas cause emotional, physical, and mental distress. Post-traumatic stress disorder is commonly associated with big *T* traumas. But ongoing exposure to little *t* traumas, especially during the developmental years, can cause significant harm to our physical, emotional, and mental development.

Little *t* traumas can stack up over time, feeling like death to our souls by a thousand paper cuts compared to one knife wound from a capital *T* trauma. But both can disrupt the organization and function of a healthy brain, negatively affect the health of our body, and fracture the soul, making it hard for us to think things that are true, honorable, just, pure, and lovely.

How many smaller adversities in life have you pushed down, believing you needed to suck it up and quit complaining? As it turns out, ignoring the effects of a hurtful event brings more pain to every part of you: physical, mental, emotional, relational, and spiritual.

Ignoring the effects of a hurtful event brings
more pain to every part of you.

While post-traumatic stress disorder is often linked to big *T* trauma, all trauma can produce long-term effects:

- denial or minimizing of event(s)
- numbness (emotions detached from thoughts and actions)
- intense anger or sorrow
- emotional outbursts
- shame about the event
- problems sleeping; insomnia
- breathing problems
- gastrointestinal problems
- high blood pressure or cardiovascular disease
- substance abuse (including food)[3]

To be clear, trauma is not our car breaking down, missing an important meeting, or having to make a speech in public (which is still a number one fear for most people). But a broken-down car or public speaking activates our stress response. Our brains don't know the difference between the perception of and the reality of danger. It's the abundance and constant presence of stress, real or perceived, whether due to big *T*, too many little *t* traumas, or a combination, that is harmful to our bodies.

Stress weakens our immune system and corrodes the engine of our car (our brain). An overload of the stress chemicals adrenaline and cortisol can also lead to serious health conditions, such as high blood pressure, weight gain, and insomnia. In addition, stress can cause brain fog and memory problems, making it difficult to choose which road to travel.[4] Anytime our bodies are overwhelmed with stress, a healthy, integrated body-brain connection is lost. No wonder Connie mindlessly reached for the box of cookies after yelling at her son for grazing the mailbox as he drove up their driveway.

During some of our early morning training sessions, Connie and I talked about how the effects of ongoing stress on her brain were making it difficult for her to make healthy change even when she tried hard and had put a good plan into place. That is what we'll examine in the next chapter as well.

As we train through this book, keep this question at the front of your mind: When it comes to your pain, will you keep thinking the same thoughts and following the path of least resistance, or will you take your pain and direct your thoughts toward the path of a renewed mind that leads to God's peace, though it's a path of greater resistance?

Enter through the narrow gate. For wide is the gate and broad is the road that leads to destruction, and many enter through it. But small is the gate and narrow the road that leads to life, and only a few find it.

MATTHEW 7:13-14, NIV

Metabolize

Mind

1. How does knowing your brain is mechanical but your mind is the real driver of your life change the way you view your health?
2. Now that you know the difference between your brain and mind, what does God want you to do?
3. In your life, would you say you've experienced more little *t* or capital *T* traumas? How do you think these events have affected your physical and emotional health (see list on page 69)?

Mouth

God, nothing about me is unknown to You. None of my days were hidden from You either. You have been there with me through all the little ts and capital Ts. You know how the pain of those moments has negatively affected my body and my brain. I believe You have purpose for my pain. I now give myself wholeheartedly to You—body, mind, and soul. Come and cleanse my body from the lies that lead my brain to backfire, causing myself and others pain. Father, heal my body and brain by filling my mind with more of You. Amen.

Move

Do the Be Still and Be Loved meditation found at https://www.revelation wellness.org/tbr/still/, which directly correlates with this chapter and the information you just read. Journal any words, visuals, or revelations you receive during your time of stillness. Then carve out twenty minutes to move your body and listen to the audio that goes along with this chapter, which you'll find at https://www.revelationwellness.org/tbr/move/.

CHAPTER 7

WHERE PAIN GOES IN YOUR BRAIN

RECENTLY I TAUGHT MY DAUGHTER, Sophia, how to drive. (And all the parents unite in one deep breath, acknowledging the heroism of my painful feat.) The first time Sophia jumped into the driver's seat, claiming her authority behind the steering wheel, she instinctively placed her right foot on the gas pedal and her left foot on the brake. She was surprised when I told her the first thing she needed to know before turning on the car was that driving an automatic vehicle requires only one of her two feet.

"That's so weird. Why can't I use both feet?" Sophia replied.

"Because—options. When driving, you want to limit them because sometimes you'll have to make quick decisions. You will choose to turn left or right. Go faster or slower. Stop or go. You don't need to drive scared, but you do need to drive totally present to the moment so you don't put yourself or another in harm's way. When you or another driver make a mistake, you will feel panic and emotionally flooded to make a decision. In that moment, your thoughts and feelings can be pulling you into two different directions. Too many options make it hard to decide. That's why your final decisions will be made through one foot, not two."

Refining and retraining our whole selves to move toward one destination is how we stay with God or, to put it another way, how we maintain oneness with God. And oneness with God is wholeness—all things working as they should, in one accord. Before the Israelites moved into the Promised Land, Moses passed on this foundational truth: "Hear, O Israel: The LORD our God, the LORD is one" (Deuteronomy 6:4). God is not distracted by adversaries or adversity, and He never runs scared in many directions as we sometimes do.

When we decide to move physically, we do it with our whole self. We can't decide to go for a run and leave our left foot, will, or emotions at home. Wherever we go, the wholeness (or whole mess) of us goes along. Our brains have an operating system that connects all parts of our bodies to help us get where we want to go and do what we want to do. It's called our nervous system.

The reason we notice we are thirsty and then walk to the kitchen, grab a glass, fill it with water, and take a sip is because our brain-body connection is hardwired with this incredibly intelligent and sophisticated communication system. It's designed to help us turn our thoughts and feelings into actions to get us what we want and where we want to go. Our nervous system is organized into two parts: central and autonomic. The central nervous system (CNS) is the wiring of nerves between the brain and the spinal cord. The CNS makes it possible for us to express ourselves through physical movement and speech. Without our CNS, we couldn't get out of bed, drive to the gym, and lift weights.

The more subtle part is the autonomic nervous system (ANS), which is perhaps even more integral but often overlooked. The ANS regulates our involuntary body functions—things we don't need to think about doing, they just get done. This includes swallowing, blinking, breathing, heart rate, respiratory rate, blood flow, pupil dilation, and digestion. Without these hidden, involuntary actions occurring, the more noticeable work of speaking, moving, and lifting weights couldn't be done.

To strengthen our body-brain connections, we must first recognize that the autonomic nervous system is comprised of two parts: the sympathetic and the parasympathetic nervous systems. The sympathetic nervous system

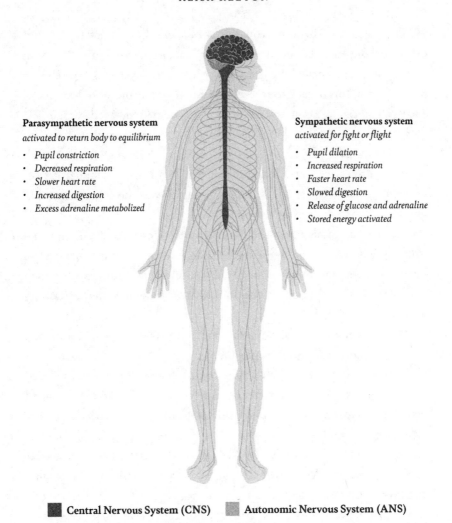

Parasympathetic nervous system
activated to return body to equilibrium

- *Pupil constriction*
- *Decreased respiration*
- *Slower heart rate*
- *Increased digestion*
- *Excess adrenaline metabolized*

Sympathetic nervous system
activated for fight or flight

- *Pupil dilation*
- *Increased respiration*
- *Faster heart rate*
- *Slowed digestion*
- *Release of glucose and adrenaline*
- *Stored energy activated*

■ **Central Nervous System (CNS)**   ■ **Autonomic Nervous System (ANS)**

enables "fight or flight" while the parasympathetic gives us the ability to "rest and digest."

The sympathetic nervous system drives our stress response: the release of cortisol and other stress hormones when we perceive a threat to our safety. This makes it possible for us to react quickly to protect ourselves. If we spot a wild-looking dog on the loose while out on a walk, our brain will take in that information and engage our sympathetic nervous system so our bodies spring into action to keep us safe.[1]

The parasympathetic nervous system enables our bodies to rest and digest, restore, and reason. If you've ever watched the ocean waves crash on the shore and smelled the salty air as you experienced an overwhelming sense of calm, this part of your nervous system was involved in that experience. When our parasympathetic nervous system is engaged, we are less likely to make fearful or hasty decisions. If the parasympathetic nervous system dominates our response to a traumatic situation, our body will go into a protective freeze mode rather than fight or flee. Think of your sympathetic nervous system as the gas pedal for your body, and the parasympathetic nervous system as your brake.

I think we can all agree, the pace of our modern world isn't slowing, which only feeds our bodies' sense that we need to live at a frenetic pace. But if we are going to move out of survival mode and stop making snap judgments that lead us to choose "quick fixes" (like bingeing or starving ourselves), we will need to strengthen our autonomic nervous system so we can slow down, hit the brake, think, and reason. Then we will know when it's time to put our foot on the gas and go.

Our body works best with an unstressed, focused, and sober-minded driver behind the wheel, one that refuses to drive the body and brain with a lead foot or stay stuck in Park on the side of the road. We can become observant drivers of our body who know when it's time to focus, punch the gas, or ease up and push on the brake. We can become sober and make better decisions as we practice ways of tuning into our ANS, which is exactly what the Move activities at the end of each chapter are doing.

Animals have nervous systems too, but they seem to process stress instinctively and much more quickly than humans. When animals are in danger, their stress response kicks in, and they do whatever needs to be done to survive. Some animals face their opponent and fight. Some run and flee. Others fall over and play dead, hoping their attacker will lose interest and leave them alone. Once the threat passes, their nervous systems automatically shift from sympathetic mode or a dominating parasympathetic mode (fight, flight, or freeze) into the parasympathetic rest and recovery mode. They do so through a variety of methods, including gentle trembling, shaking, taking deep breaths, sweating, and even reenacting some aggressive fight behaviors. Psychologist Peter Levine calls this discharge, a process by which the animal automatically resets itself to a stress-free state. Animals that don't discharge are more likely to die.[2]

Wait a minute: Trembling, shaking, taking deep breaths, sweating, and reenacting behaviors help an animal reset? Those things sound a lot like what happens in any Revelation Fitness class I teach. In chapter 12, you will learn more about how exercise improves our brains, strengthens our nervous systems, and helps us when we feel stuck in a cycle of fight, flight, or freeze. Until then, keep training with me in the Metabolize portions of this book!

Now, of course, we are not animals. We are the children of God—the apex, the high point of His creation on earth. Men and women were made in God's image; animals were not. As a result, we humans have bodies with the power and potential to create, make meaning out of life, and do things animals will never be able to do. Like animals, our bodies are fully present to the adversity we experience, but unlike animals, we don't automatically unload and discharge our stress. We tend to hold the adversity inside until we find a way to release it—to shift from fight, flight, or freeze to rest and recovery. Some people find safe and healthy means to discharge their distress, while others turn to destructive ways. Some people go for walks and talk while others run and numb.

I believe that God wants us to be able to shake off our hurt, but unlike animals, He wants to be with us and help us to do it with Him. God wants us to move on from the past without forgetting what we've learned. That's because every difficult moment offers us the opportunity to make our hearts, minds, bodies, and lives look more like Christ's. Becoming more like Him pleases our Father's heart and is our spiritual act of worship (Romans 12:1-2). The more we look like Christ, the better the world sees Him and the more our Father will be glorified and known.

Every difficult moment offers us the opportunity to look more like Christ. The more we look like Christ, the more the world sees Him and our Father is glorified and known.

No challenging moment surprises God. He has signed off on every moment of your life, and each is designed to help conform you more into the image of Christ. Let's be people who trust God with our pain, who go to Him to stay loose and shake off our stress, rather than people who stay rigid and blame God for our adversity. We will encounter troubles, but we can be quick to metabolize our pain by going to God. This is how we prevent pain from having the last word and make it useful for God's glory.

Adversity comes with a gift, the potential for us to have greater intimacy *with* God and become more Christlike. We just need to know the Way to drive our car (our body) to get there.

Driving to the High or Low Places

On Saturday mornings, I like to lace up my trail shoes and head for the closest mountain. The sound of dirt and loose shale crunching under my feet as I propel myself onward and upward gives me life. In all my years of hiking, I've never traveled a perfectly straight trail to the top. The rocky path under my feet always zig-zags and undulates. Little by little, one forceful breath and step at a time, I arrive at my high-point destination. It's on a mountaintop that I gain something that's hard to get on the valley floor. Perspective.

One thing I certainly didn't have in my youth was perspective, defined as "the capacity to view things in their true relations or relative importance."[3] Back then, I thought the entire world revolved around me—and most of my peers thought the same thing. Our brains do not reach full development until we reach our midtwenties.[4] Isn't it interesting that it isn't until we have passed through the most formative years of our lives—infancy, childhood, adolescence, and young adulthood—that we have a fully formed brain? This certainly explains some of the foolish and half-brained decisions I made concerning fashion, fun, and friends.

For simplicity's sake, let's learn about our brains by considering its two parts: the bottom and the top. Or better yet, the valley floor and the mountaintop.

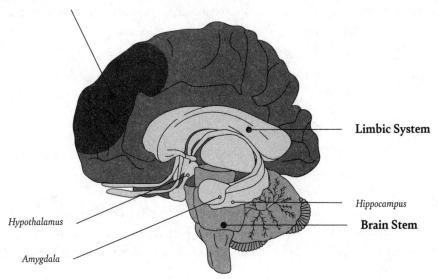

Medial prefrontal cortex

Limbic System

Hippocampus

Brain Stem

Hypothalamus

Amygdala

The valley floor

Take the palm of your left hand and place it behind your head at the base of your skull. If your hand were holding your brain, you would be cradling the brain stem and parts of your limbic system. We will call this our valley floor. Our brain stem is the earliest part of the brain to develop in our mother's womb and is the only part of our brain fully developed at birth. It controls functions like breathing, blinking, swallowing, heart rate, blood pressure, and the transition from wakefulness to sleep. It's responsible for the actions of basic survival—like our autonomic nervous system, it controls things your body will do without you telling it to do them.

Our limbic system comes next and is connected to our brain stem and continues to develop after birth. It is responsible for motivation and emotions, and it even stores the memory of our emotions. Inside our limbic brain is the amygdala, which helps govern our emotions and connects memories to our emotions. The amygdala is a cluster of neurons shaped like an almond that acts like a smoke detector.[5] Whenever you perceive a threat, your amygdala is alarmed and communicates to the brain's hypothalamus,

"FIRE! FIRE! FIRE!" The hypothalamus then activates the autonomic nervous system. Like a personal bodyguard that's been with you from birth, the ANS has three takedown moves: fight, flight, or freeze.[6]

- *Fight*: You employ all systems of your body and the energy of your emotions to fight the source of threat.
- *Flight*: You gather up all your energy and run away as fast as possible from the source of threat.
- *Freeze*: Your nervous system is overwhelmed, and you feel helpless. You freeze.

Basic survival instincts come from these early developed, lower parts of the structure of your brain[7] while your ability to think, reason, and think of yourself and others with compassion, kindness, and empathy come from a higher place.

The mountaintop

Take the palm of your right hand and place it over your forehead. Behind your skull in this area of your brain is what's known as the medial prefrontal cortex (MPFC). It is responsible for our memory, attention, decision-making, and reasoning. In *The Body Keeps the Score*, psychiatrist Bessel van der Kolk calls this part of the brain the watchtower.[8] The MPFC enables you to remain calm, cool, and collected even when the smoke detector of your amygdala tries to hijack a moment, telling you to fight, flee, or freeze. In a moment of stress, we are inclined to take quick shelter in the valley floor of our brains rather than remain in the high and safe place.

The objective of all war is to subdue and overcome your enemy. Taking higher ground is advantageous because it enables you to see what's going on in surrounding territory. You can see where your enemies are and what snares, bombs, or traps they've set. The most dangerous place to be during combat is in a valley, since these wide-open spaces have few places to hide from your enemy. Of course, taking high ground is much harder than staying down. When we are let down by life or hurt by others, it's easiest to stay on the valley floor of our limbic brain, freaking out and running in circles either fighting or fleeing from our enemy. We often don't stop to consider the high place in our brain—our MPFC, the area of our brain responsible for higher reasoning.[9]

When we love and think optimistically, we stimulate our MPFC. In fact, the more we think hopeful and loving thoughts, the more we stimulate and strengthen this area of our brain. In this way our brain can be trained and stimulated for growth, just like a muscle. Dr. Caroline Leaf, a research neuroscientist, mental health expert, and believer in Christ, notes that "Our brains are made for love. Not fear. Not performance. Not aggression. But LOVE."[10] It seems God designed our brains to work best in the presence of love and not fear, and our physical body benefits from the positive energy of love and optimistic thinking that originate in the mountaintop of our brain, our MPFC.

God designed our brains to work best in
the presence of love and not fear.

Like soldiers on the battlefield, our minds have a watchtower, a high place to run to when the first bomb of adversity goes off, but how will we know to go there if nobody has ever shown us the way? Reading this book and completing the Metabolize sections will help you find it!

When deciding what to eat, how to move, or what we think about our bodies, we will do a better job with a stronger and more activated MPFC. Using reasoning in our thinking provides us with a 360-degree view to observe our circumstances and respond to our emotions calmly rather than erratically as we would in the valley. As Christ followers, we are not to be reactors but responders—just like Jesus, who never ran yelling into the streets, blaming everyone who did Him wrong or running from His Pharisaic haters.

But because our MPFCs are not fully developed until we reach our mid-twenties, it's easy to see why growing brains affected by adversity tend to respond with fear and shame. They then encode this pattern in their neurons in an attempt to survive and stay safe. But now that God is here with us and in us, it's time to carve out a new path, the way of Christ. When He came to earth, His body endured emotional aches and physical pains just as ours do.

We, the people of God, have a stronger and higher mountaintop than our MPFC alone. We have access to God, high and lifted up, seated in the heavenly places with a 360-degree view over the tactics of our enemy. He is with us in every battle we face, whether it's moving the number on the scale under our feet or responding to a negative report from our doctor. God, our Father, is our watchtower. In love, He calls us higher, to Himself, and gives us the ability to reason.

David drew on the strength of God and called Him his high place when he was being pursued by his enemies.

> The LORD is my rock, and my fortress, and my deliverer; my God,
> my strength, in whom I will trust; my buckler, and the horn of
> my salvation, and my high tower.
>
> PSALM 18:2, KJV

The pain we carry encodes a path in our brain that will keep us stuck in the valley, driven primarily by the amygdala and hypothalamus. In fact, the reasons you overeat or undernourish, obsess about your body or neglect it, may have something to do with how long you've been living with an overactive limbic brain.

When you purposely get into your body, either to move, sweat, and breathe, or to be still and meditate on God's Word, you're allowing the Holy Spirit to use His power to discharge you from the valley floor. He can get you to the mountaintop, help you take the high ground, and bring you to the high tower where you can meet with God. In His presence, you can receive fresh perspective and revelation of the battle that's taking place in your valley floor—the place of learned memory and emotion stored in your brain.

When we operate from the low places of our brain, we tend to think, feel, and choose as we did in our youth, believing no one is going to help us and lacking the rational response of a fully formed brain. Yet, because of Christ, we are new creations with renewed minds and redeemed bodies.

Therefore, if anyone is in Christ, the new creation has come: The old has gone, the new is here!

2 CORINTHIANS 5:17, NIV

In Christ, we are new creations who think, say, and do new things, even when we feel the pull toward something old, like fear or shame.

New creations refuse to hang their heads and wait for a validating number on the scale or for that elusive moment when they will look in the mirror and finally love what they see. New creations live with God; they walk, talk, and sit with Him as they strive to live for something more than what they can see. New creations know that it's from the unseen that seen things come to be. New creations know they are now in Christ, with access to the high tower of His compassion, love, and reasoning.

Metabolize

Mind

1. Are you more likely to use the gas pedal (fight or flight) or the brakes (freeze)? Why?
2. What are some of the thoughts and behaviors you fall back into when you're on the valley floor?
3. Describe what it would be like for you to live with a body that thinks, feels, and chooses from a mountaintop perspective. How would your life be different?

Mouth

Place your left hand behind your head at the base of your skull and the right hand over your forehead as you pray.

Holy Spirit, my brain needs Your healing power. I repent for thinking that I or my body is broken. The pain I've lived through has affected my brain. I have been able to survive, but now I want to thrive. Come and cleanse my brain of its pain, whether it started in my youth or yesterday. Connect my limbic brain to my reasoning brain as You originally designed them. And give me the grace to do the things I need to do to partner with the restoration of my mind and my brain. In the healing name of Jesus I ask these things. Amen.

Move

Take ten minutes to listen to this Be Still and Be Loved meditation: https://www.revelationwellness.org/tbr/still/.

Sometime before you move on to the next chapter, lace up your shoes and go for twenty minutes of movement while listening to this: https://www.revelationwellness.org/tbr/move/.

CHAPTER 8

TENSION VS. PAIN

IF I WERE TO SURVEY THE PEOPLE IN my fitness classes, the majority of them would agree that the first five to ten minutes of a training session are the most uncomfortable. When we move our bodies, we feel resistance. That comes from the tension—the burning of energy—we exert as we push against a force. Some people want to be more physically active but struggle to make a habit of moving their bodies because they can't get past the mental hump of the discomfort caused during the first few minutes of exercise. How I wish they knew that, once we're moving, we get swept up into a state that feels like flow.

In fact, doctors encourage people who feel stressed to exercise because during physical activity, the muscle tightness and tension we carry in our bodies, due to stress, can be positively released. When we exercise, our muscles contract and lengthen repeatedly, leaving us with a sense of slack in our bodies by the end of physical activity. Most people would agree that engaging and releasing tension by moving our bodies, like going for a brisk walk, is a better choice for dealing with stress than punching a hole in the wall, shouting in someone's face, or turning to a couple glasses of wine. By the way, stress isn't bad in itself. Stress gets us to focus and helps us do work. But stress (or tension) should come and it should go.

Our intention in part 1, The Warm-Up, has been to learn how pain has interrupted our desire for God and, biologically, has left a mark on our bodies and brains. As we wrap up this first section, I hope you are beginning to feel fired up and are energized to keep going. It can be uncomfortable to recognize and confront the effects of pain, so I commend you for doing the hard work needed to deal with them.

The truth is, we can't escape all stress because everything God created on earth exists in tension. While we feel resistance in our bodies while running intervals or lifting weights, that tension exists outside of us as well. For instance, my husband and I have had to navigate many moments of tension over the past twenty-five years. In many ways we are so opposite of one another. This opposition creates tension between us. We were created differently on purpose because our distinctives reflect the beauty and artistry of God's creation, which emerged with the creation of Adam and Eve.

> God created man in his own image, in the image of God he created him; male and female he created them. And God blessed them. And God said to them, "Be fruitful and multiply and fill the earth and *subdue* it, and have *dominion* over the fish of the sea and over the birds of the heavens and over every living thing that moves on the earth."
>
> GENESIS 1:27-28 (EMPHASIS MINE)

These last two directives from God—to subdue and have dominion—are significant if we are going to process our pain while living in a world marked by tension. The Hebrew word translated "subdue" here is *kabas*, which means "to subject," "to force," "to keep under," or "to bring into bondage,"[1] and the word translated "dominion" is *rada*, which means "to rule," "to tread down," or "to scrape out."[2] Those sound like strange commands to give two people without sin who lived in a beautiful garden with

God, walking in His perfect peace. They sound instead as if they belong in the job description of a jailhouse warden tasked with breaking up scuffles between bunking inmates. Bring into bondage; tread down and scrape out. That sounds like violent work. What gives, God?

Although the Garden of Eden was a place of abundant life and peace, God didn't intend for people to live in eternal vacation mode. We were created for good work. And all work gets done through tension. Perhaps a part of this good work given to humanity was to be sure that we kept Satan and his opposing forces in their place.

We were created for good work. And all work gets done through tension.

In Genesis 1:28, God blessed Adam and Eve and told them what they were to do. God knew that Satan, in the form of a snake, would soon whisper words that sounded different from what God had told them. The devil would unleash a new type of tension, "the state of latent hostility or opposition between individuals or groups."[3] In commanding Adam and Eve to subdue and take dominion, God may have been preparing them to hold their ground—on behalf of all creation—in the presence of the forces of opposition and destruction, namely the devil.

Satan is a spiritual being who was created by God but fell into pride and became God's enemy. God sent Satan out of His presence in heaven and cast him down to earth (along with a band of other rebellious angel beings). Ever since, good and evil have pulled in opposite directions and created ongoing tension. God is the Master Artist of the world who allows His creation to exist inside the tension of two opposing forces: good and evil.

To metabolize our pain well, we need to learn how to harness tension by seeing and using opposition as God does. Resistance is an opportunity for the goodness of God to be magnified through the demonstration of His power over evil and His ability to exponentially multiply good.

The Difference between Pain and Tension

If I were to ask you to hold a five-pound weight over your head, you could do so (unless you are injured). You would feel the downward pull of the weight due to the force of gravity while your shoulder muscles continued to shorten to keep your arm up against it. You would feel the tension of the opposing forces, but you wouldn't feel pain—at least until you moved past your physical ability to endure. Then the pain would start to set in.

From the beginning, God created us for a life of tension, but never pain. Tension is not comfortable, but it also isn't pain. Peace is not the absence of tension, but the power to subdue internal and external conflict by submitting our free will—the right to think, feel, and choose whatever we want—to God's will.

God created us for a life of tension, but never pain.

Picture the moment Eve first saw the snake moving toward her. Satan's presence must have brought a felt sense of stress (tension) to her. The words "Did God really say?" would have been confusing and distressing. Perhaps Eve felt her stomach turn, her palms sweat—the result of a rush of cortisol when in the presence of Satan, God's opposing enemy.

Adam and Eve never needed to fear. God was with them as they stewarded creation. They needed to remember who they were and do what they had been told to do. To maintain rule over the earth as God's son and daughter, they needed to exercise their authority and maintain God's peace on earth.

> Now the serpent was more crafty than any other beast of the field that the LORD God had made. He said to the woman, "Did God actually say, 'You shall not eat of any tree in the garden'?" . . . But the serpent said to the woman, "You will not surely die. For God knows that when you eat of it your eyes will be opened, and you will be like God, knowing good and evil."
>
> GENESIS 3:1, 4-5

When tempted, Eve should have told Satan, "Wait a minute. What you're saying is making me feel different from what I felt when God spoke. It is causing me tension; it's confusing me. It doesn't sound like what we've heard. We are going to go talk to God again, and then we will come back and deal with you." At that, the serpent would have slithered away. When we stay with God and His Word, no matter how conflicted or confused we feel in that tension, we are subduing and keeping dominion.

Unfortunately, Adam and Eve didn't use their free will to hold their ground, to stand on what God had said. When faced with the tension of temptation, they gave in. They fell for the lie that God was holding out on them and that being like God would satisfy their wonder and curiosity. Instead of going to their Father in the tension, with their stress—their turning stomachs and sweaty palms, their questions and curiosities—they gave time, attention, and credence to a "creeping thing."

Adam and Eve's curiosity about their new home and their misuse of free will led them to disobey God's command, which caused them to forfeit the key to their home in the Garden of Eden. Satan had begun his mission of roaming the earth looking for image bearers of God to kill, steal, and destroy. Because humanity gave in to the tension of temptation—a failure to keep the forces of evil at bay—pain entered the world. And all of God's creation, which had been placed under the dominion of humanity, was affected.

> To the woman [God] said, "I will surely multiply your pain in childbearing; in *pain* you shall bring forth children. Your desire will be contrary to your husband, but he shall rule over you."
> GENESIS 3:16 (EMPHASIS MINE)

> And to Adam he said, "Because you have listened to the voice of your wife and have eaten of the tree of which I commanded you, 'You shall not eat of it,' cursed is the ground because of you; in *pain* you shall eat of it all the days of your life; thorns and thistles it shall bring forth for you."
> GENESIS 3:17-18 (EMPHASIS MINE)

We ache for a body that doesn't age, a beauty that never fades, and a love that never ends because we are all trying to get back home to the Garden. We want to live in our bodies without pain. And in our desire for no pain, we cause more pain when we try to live without God.

Strength through Resistance

In fitness, we often use resistance tubing to tone and strengthen our muscles. The key to getting the most out of these glorified rubber bands is to secure one end of the tube using a fixed anchor point (like around a doorknob or under your foot) while stretching the tube and performing proper range of motion for a given muscle. Each repetition of movement against the tube's changing resistance stimulates the muscle fiber and, if done consistently, leads to muscle growth. But ask anyone who has used one of these torture tubes before what they fear, and they'll tell you that it's hearing the dreaded *snap!* followed by a high-pitched *slap!* That is the sound of high-velocity rubber breaking force on human skin. My body still bears the marks left by suddenly untethered tubes.

Likewise sin snaps the cord of loving-kindness between us and God, and—*whap!*—pain is the result. Next we feel shame, and we wander even further from God's loving-kindness, tethering ourselves to things of this world that without God's purposes behind them, can oppose God and be used for evil. Things we think will satisfy—relationships, sex, money, beauty, influence, and fame—are misplaced desires that only cause and compound the *whap!* of more pain.

When temptation overwhelms us, it's usually because we couldn't handle one more moment under the stress, the tension. It's too much to handle and all we want is relief, especially if our stress-response brain is pulling up old memories and constructs, which are designed to jump into action to keep us safe. So we give in to Satan's bidding for things like comfort food, drugs, alcohol, sex, or the perfect body. The tension of temptation isn't sin. Giving into temptation is sin. And sin causes pain.

Yet God is bigger than our sin, bigger than our pain. Even before He announced His judgment on Adam and Eve, God cursed the serpent. Not only that, but He also promised Satan that from Adam and Eve's offspring would come one who would "crush your head" (Genesis 3:15, NIV). Think of that! Even before God had confronted Adam and Eve for their sin, He had planned a way to free us from the tension and pain caused by sin.

God is not opposed to conflict. If He were, He would never have created Satan. In God's mysterious ways on earth, opposition can lead to something exceedingly and abundantly better than if there were no evil and only good. In the days ahead, and if not already, you will undoubtedly face the stress of opposition. At some point, you will get sick. When feeling your strongest, you may get injured. Your job might demand more of you than you would like to give, leaving you less time to hit the gym, or go for a walk, to unwind your muscle tension. Or you will get distracted by an image you see on your phone that doesn't look like the one you see in your mirror. When those moments show up, subdue and keep dominion. Remember whose image you bear, the One who stands in opposition to the evil one, who enjoys stressing you out with what you perceive as bad news. Like resistance to a muscle, whatever is coming against you is there to increase your knowledge of God, His truth, and His love. It's for these moments in life we train.

Over and over in Scripture, God speaks of His desire to reestablish fellowship with us. For instance, God continually pursued the rebellious, idolatrous people of Israel, despite their continued attempts to find life apart from Him: "I led them with cords of kindness, with the bands of love, and I became to them as one who eases the yoke on their jaws, and I bent down to them and fed them" (Hosea 11:4).

God's loving-kindness is like a cord that tethers us to His unceasing love. He pursues us when we wander away in our desire for an earthly beauty that never fades or a body that never quits. He is the One who created all things and still holds them together in creative tension. We can be sure that, as we begin to actively process our pain in the next stage, The Workout, God's mercy and grace will hold us fast.

Metabolize

Mind

1. How do you know the difference between tension and pain in your body? (Try to explain the difference in terms of how they feel.)

2. Think through your daily routine. What times bring the most stress or tension? What would life in your body be like if you could subdue (bring to order) and keep dominion (take out the trash)?
3. How does knowing that before sin entered the world, God created the world with tension (the presence of opposition) change the way you view your pain?

Mouth

God, You are a good Father, and all You create is good. You hold everything together inside a holy tension. Please come and help me recognize that tension is not pain and that when tension shows up, Your cords of loving-kindness enable me to stay with You in Your perfect peace rather than seek to survive on my own. Heal my mind, Father. Heal my brain. Make my body the perfect place to host Your presence and hold Your holy tension so I might multiply good, as well as subdue and keep dominion. Amen.

Move

Use this link for your Kind-Mind Renewing Movement: https://www.revelationwellness.org/tbr/move/.

Use this link for the Be Still and Be Loved meditation that goes along with this chapter: https://www.revelationwellness.org/tbr/still/.

The Workout

Expressing Your Energy

But when he came to himself, he said, "How many
of my father's hired servants have more than
enough bread, but I perish here with hunger!"

LUKE 15:17

CHAPTER 9

FEELING YOUR FEELINGS

YOUR BODY AND BRAIN ARE FOR YOU.

Whether you have lived through catastrophic, painful events or small, steady stresses that never seem to end, your body has done its best to keep you alive. Your brain makes order from what feels out of your control, and your body responds to its directives.

The first part of this book, The Warm-Up, was all about understanding what has been happening inside your body and brain due to the challenges you've faced. Now it's time to begin the The Workout section. These chapters will show you how to confront and work on anything that inhibits your healing.

As we move into stage 3, Expressing Your Energy, please know this: Much of the difficulty in making good choices around your health and well-being is due to the schemes of Satan, your enemy. Planting suspicions against God and temptations to sin into your mind is his game. Sin has negatively affected your body-brain connection, but you can retrain your body and brain to agree with the mind of Christ as you follow the Spirit's leading. The first step is to recognize and befriend your body's emotions, feelings, and felt sense.

Imagine you are taking a leisurely stroll after dinner. As you turn a corner, you notice a large dog running free with his tail and ears down, headed straight toward you. Your body tenses and your eyes widen as you feel a rush of helplessness and alarm. In just an instant, your body's emotions, feelings, and felt sense have all been activated.

Let's consider the distinction between emotions and feelings. Emotions can arise before you even form a thought; they are a survival feature of your body-brain wiring system. Six basic emotions—happiness, sadness, anger, fear, surprise, and disgust—can be triggered subconsciously.[1] In the case of the dog running free, your body senses a threat and responds with fear before you've fully processed what is happening. Feelings, on the other hand, are something you become conscious of as you ascribe nuance and meaning to a particular emotion. As the dog charges toward you, you recognize feelings of powerlessness and terror.

Think of emotions as six big Igloo water coolers holding different sports drinks, each containing ingredients that account for the different tastes. Feelings are the ingredients inside the water cooler of each emotion, and they describe in more detail the bigger emotion you are having. When you tell someone "I am mad," they probably have a sense of what you mean even though they will never know exactly how you are feeling. Feelings are personal. Two people can experience the same emotion but have different feelings. On a deeper lever, feelings produce what is called a felt sense in your body.

The ability to recognize what's going on in your body is called interoception. And here's a great reason to be in touch with your body's sensations: A person with strong interoceptive awareness is more likely to be successful as an intuitive eater. This type of eater eats when they are hungry and stops when they are full, so they feel no need to diet. They also enjoy moving their body because it feels good. This felt sense is the most subtle part of your emotional life. You and I don't often take time to recognize what our body is experiencing while in the throes of feeling an emotion. As a big dog sprints toward you, you may find yourself sweating and breathing faster as your body prepares to run or to crouch down in a defensive posture. During times of distress, getting in touch with your felt sense can help you befriend your body as the ally it is.

*Getting in touch with your felt sense can help
you befriend your body as the ally it is.*

Here's another example of how the three parts of experiencing an emotion may play out: You are angry at Angela (an emotion), frustrated (a feeling) because she didn't turn her work in on time, and a warm sensation (a felt sense) fills your face.

Here are some other words you might use to describe a felt sense in your body:

- dense
- breathless
- fluttery
- tingly

- hot
- cold
- buzzy
- constricted

- weighty
- sweaty
- bubbly
- achy

Why does this matter? Learning to identify feelings is important for everyone, especially people who have experienced trauma:

> Trauma generates emotions, and unless you process these
> emotions at the time they occur, they can become stuck in
> your system, negatively affecting you both psychologically
> and physically. The healthy flow and processing of distressing
> emotions like anger, sadness, grief and fear are all essential. You
> will never resolve underlying issues if you deny and run from
> your feelings. Suppressed emotions don't just go away; instead
> they become toxic.[2]

When we deny our emotions and feelings, our health can suffer and we may be hindered from growing into Christlikeness. That's because feelings pushed down inside can make us sick or explode out of us like weapons we use to protect ourselves and harm others.

Though my mom used food to push down her emotions, she often expressed her feelings quite freely. As a child, then, I understood that expressing what I was feeling was not against the rules in our household. My mother was a feeling artist who used her emotions as a palette, her feelings for paint, and her body as her brush. Dark colors splashed onto my brother and me on her painful days. And then there were the bright and colorful days when she pushed down her pain and encouraged lots of silly play. During those times, I remember her grabbing my hand, cranking up the local Top 40 radio station, and bopping around the den with me. Her example taught me to display my feelings just as spontaneously as she did.

Perhaps the emotional environment you grew up in wasn't as colorful and messy as mine. Perhaps your family kept their feelings under tight control so that your home environment was tidier and neater with no wet paint allowed. Perhaps keeping calm and carrying on represented intelligence and nobility.

Regardless, feelings are not to be feared, smashed down, and compressed, nor are they to be used to manipulate, scare, or oppress others. God gave you feelings to help you know where you are at all times in relationship to His presence and peace. Just as a star on a map at an amusement park map says "you are here," so you know how to find your way to the enchanted castle, feelings tell you where you are in relationship to God and His Kingdom. And feelings help you know what you need when you are tempted by your enemy. If the emotion of sadness is followed by a feeling of loneliness, you can sense the heaviness in your chest and go to God for comfort and companionship. Or you can reach out and call a friend. Feeling your feelings and going to God is one way you "take heart" whenever you face trouble: "In the world you will have tribulation. But take heart; I have overcome the world" (John 16:33).

Next time you are tempted to ridicule your body, feel disgust at what you see in the mirror, or plunge into another diet routine that will change

God gave you feelings to help you know where you are at all times in relationship to His presence and peace.

only the shape of your body and not your heart, take heart! You're experiencing feelings and an underlying emotion—energy in motion.

Give yourself permission to feel your feelings. Just remember that they are given to be felt, not done. You are free to feel emotions; you just don't want them to eclipse your desire for God or take you from His presence.

Drop the star to pinpoint where you are in relationship to God's heart and His Kingdom. Gather up what feels like your mess and take it to God. He's not disgusted by your tangled emotions. So that you can find wholeness, He requires that you hand over your whole mess.

When Emotions Rule

Let's go back to the beginning and look at the role that emotions played in Eve's response to the serpent.

> When the woman saw that the tree was good for food, and that
> it was a delight to the eyes, and that the tree was to be desired
> to make one wise, she took of its fruit and ate, and she also gave
> some to her husband who was with her, and he ate. Then the eyes
> of both were opened, and they knew that they were naked. And
> they sewed fig leaves together and made themselves loincloths.
> GENESIS 3:6-7

Though originally designed to walk in perfect peace with God as they experienced awe and wonder in a beautiful garden, Adam and Eve chose to pull away from their Creator. At the suggestion of their enemy, they ate the forbidden fruit and immediately went from experiencing positively charged feelings of love, joy, and peace to viewing their bodies wrongly and feeling shame over their nakedness. When they gave in to temptation, they snapped the cord of God's loving-kindness. Separated from God, they were mad, sad, and scared for the first time.

Mad: Adam and Eve's anger showed up as they tried to shift blame from themselves and on to each other (Genesis 3:12-13). I don't know about you, but when I am angry, I am always looking for someone to blame.

Bad: Adam and Eve knew they were guilty of doing something they shouldn't have done. They felt bad and tried to hide. Bad brings with it the feeling of shame. Because of it, Adam and Eve saw themselves differently from the way God had. With their knowledge of good and evil (something they were never meant to know, which is why God asked them not to eat from that tree), they no longer saw their bodies as God did. They no longer saw them as good and complete but as something to hide with fig leaves.

Sad: When Adam and Eve received the consequences for doing what they shouldn't have done, they felt sorrow. Eve was told that she would experience physical pain in childbearing and that her desire would be for her husband, who would not meet all her needs. And Adam would now experience frustration and pain as he worked to multiply good from the ground. Experiencing a life with pain would be a shared sad experience for Adam and Eve.

Fear: Instead of feeling excited at the sound of God's voice, Adam and Eve feared what would happen when God found out what they had done. They ran away from Him and tried to hide. Their fear must have increased once they were evicted from the only home they had ever known, the Garden of Eden (which means "pleasure" or "delight"). Angels, who flashed flaming swords and guarded the tree of life, sent them away from the pleasure of God's presence to journey into an unruly and unknown land. God's presence would no longer feel as near as it once had. And so Adam and Eve began wandering, searching, and desiring the pleasures they'd lost, which had been replaced by emotional chaos inside their bodies.

If we trace negative feelings back to their origin, we end back at the mad, bad, sad, or scared feelings that showed up when humans first sinned. The ongoing presence of these negatively charged emotions contribute to ongoing stress, stunt the healthy body-brain connection, and negatively affect our bodies, particularly our immune systems.[3]

We feel before we think.[4] Before we were old enough to use our thoughts to connect words to form sentences about our needs, we had emotions, feelings, and a felt sense. This may help explain why some people turn to food when flooded with emotions. We are inclined to do our feelings before we think about them. Our experience of pain is tightly intertwined with an emotion. In fact, research shows it's possible for a baby to experience pain in utero, which means people can experience pain long before they have the words to explain what they are feeling.[5]

We are inclined to do our feelings
before we think about them.

I like to refer to mad, bad, sad, and scared as the four warhorses of our emotions. They are trained to keep us alive and safe. They hear the battle cry (our amygdala), then swiftly show up to sweep us off our feet. They scoop us up and throw us on their backs, galloping toward our hideout or charging the front lines so we can confront any threat head-on. The four horses never show up to take us on a leisurely horseback ride down by the stream when we are in pain *unless* we have trained them to do so.

We want these warhorses to come to our aid if there is an actual war. But we must remember that we own them—we own our feelings of mad, bad, sad, and scared. With God's help, we can subdue and take dominion over these horses of harmful feelings, receiving His wholeness in exchange for our whole mess of feelings.

If we lack love, joy, or peace, we can know that we're being tempted to trust in something or someone other than God. Our minds wandered to a place where God didn't lead. Or perhaps we were dragged by a wild horse because we didn't keep dominion over it.

Because God is the author and overseer of creation, our mad, bad, sad, and scared feelings come as no surprise to Him. However, we shouldn't ignore the energy these emotions create because, as we learned in chapter 3, energy can't be destroyed; it can only be transmitted to someone or transformed into something else. With God's help and through His Word stored in our hearts, we can take negative feelings to God, hold them up to what He says, and then watch as He changes negative emotions into positive energy.

The Simplicity of Sadness

Before we end this chapter, let's focus on the emotion of sad. Unlike mad, bad, and scared, sad is unique. It doesn't charge out with the same type of weaponry or protection as mad, bad, and scared. When we are mad, we can fight and blame. When we feel bad, we can hide behind something (as Adam and Eve did when they made loincloth from fig leaves). And when we are scared, our sympathetic nervous system can strengthen our legs and arms so we can run and flee. But sad is sad. It neither compels us to hide nor compels us to fight with weaponry. Yet sadness still has energy, even if it feels tiny and unseen. In fact, that seed of energy holds a secret superpower that mad, bad, and scared people lack. God says He is especially near to those who are sad:

> The LORD is close to the brokenhearted
> and saves those who are crushed in spirit.
> PSALM 34:18, NIV

> You're blessed when you're at the end of your rope. With less of
> you there is more of God and his rule.
> MATTHEW 3:5, MSG

Perhaps God finds it easier to come near because we aren't busy running away, hiding, or fighting with the wrong weaponry. I pray you take any sad energy, transforming it into power that moves you closer to God's heart because He is near you.

Now that we live "east of Eden," feelings are complicated, but God remains the same. Instead of condemning ourselves for what we feel or don't feel, let's become curious so we can move toward a more empathetic, compassionate, and healing space without judgment or shame.

God invites us to tell Him how we feel so He can tell us what He sees. When we have His perspective, our feelings operate like friends of God that encourage us to remain in His perfect love, joy, and peace. If we become more fascinated and less frustrated by our feelings, we are more likely to maintain the mind of Christ, who even when He was mocked and jeered, continued to do the next best thing.

It's not a sin to feel bad feelings, but it is a sin to act on them. When Adam and Eve were tempted, they should have gone to God to talk with Him about their confusing feelings. Jesus has made a way for us to do just that. In the presence of an enemy who shames our bodies; tells us we are fat, old, or weak; and demands that we work harder, or who tells us that God doesn't care about our bodies and we should eat anything we want, we can talk with Christ about our feelings and our needs. If there's something we need to do to exercise dominion over the four horses of mad, bad, sad, and scared, God will give us the grace and power to do it!

Jesus came to give you more than a way to heaven where you will finally get a glorious body and unending peace. Jesus came to give you a real life here on earth and to give you His abiding peace in your whole mind, heart, body, and soul. Until now, your brain and body have been doing their best to help you survive, either by running mile after mile as you beat your body into shape or by running to the pantry so you can stuff down your feelings and keep you afraid of seeing your own body.

Your feelings are never too much or too little for Jesus. Picture Him now, looking at you with His loving eyes as He extends His hand and invites you to "bring it!"

Metabolize

Mind

1. Which of the four horses (mad, bad, sad, scared) comes for you most often? What feelings are associated with that emotion? How would you describe its felt sense in your body?
2. Why is God asking you to come to Him to feel?

Mouth

God, thank You for the gift of my feelings. You gave them to me, not to ruin me, but so I might come to You in all things. I want to feel my feelings and not do them. Help me come to You with my feelings and trust You over my feelings. I want my body to contain Your perfect peace. Amen.

Move

Take ten minutes to listen to this Be Still and Be Loved meditation that goes along with what you just read: https://www.revelationwellness.org/tbr /still/. Then sometime today, lace up your shoes and go for a walk while listening to this link: https://www.revelationwellness.org/tbr/move/.

CHAPTER 10

EXTINGUISHING PAIN

"Jack, you're so invigorating!"

Sophia's screeching tone didn't match her word choice. What my daughter meant to tell her brother was "Jack, you're so infuriating!" (as in "You are bothering me!"). But in her quickness to fire a verbal heat-seeking missile, she defaulted to a like-sounding word. Instead of speaking a hurtful word, she had spoken a blessing. In that moment when Jack refused to watch another episode of *Dora the Explorer*, Sophia had been in her limbic brain, outraged and inflamed by something Jack had done to disrupt her comfort zone and sense of control.

The world would be a better place if we couldn't speak a hurtful word even if we tried, but that's not our reality. That's yet another reason we must learn to drop into our bodies to feel our feelings and deal with our overactive emotional brains.

When our comfort or control is disrupted, the emotional portion of our brain knows what to do. Bypassing our mind and ability to reason, the warhorse charges to the valley floor to fight using old weaponry, like the hurtful words we learned in previous experiences of fear, anger, and shame. In a stressful situation in which we forget to exercise dominion, our emotional brain convinces us it knows what to do—we must protect ourselves, and when the moment of crisis passes, we must soothe the ache from the aftershock.

When I am stressed, fearful, or sad, you'll never hear me say "Boy, I would love a salad right now!" Nope! When life is hard, my emotional brain screams for comfort and pleasure like a toddler who wants their way. I want to be soothed. I want pleasure. I want immediate relief.

Dopamine is the feel-good hormone of the body that motivates us into wanting pleasure and drives us into a state of pleasure when we suffer. Most people find eating enjoyable, especially when the food is tasty and easily accessible. When looking for food to offset our pain (even actual hunger pains), we often look for a quick hit of pleasure through foods with higher amounts of refined sugar, including bread, pasta, pastries, candy, and sugary drinks. Once consumed, these quick-energy foods release dopamine so we feel good. In fact, sugar has been shown to affect our brains like a line of cocaine.[1] The difference, of course, is that, unlike cocaine, sugar is legal and it's in foods we eat.

What we must become aware of is when we are seeking pleasure through food even though we are not hungry. As my client Tom once said, "Food is for daily fuel, not a daily fiesta!" Any external stimulus we use to dampen our state of pain can also dampen our body's natural ability to experience and produce pleasure. Neuroscience calls this process neuroadaptation. In her book *Dopamine Nation*, psychiatrist Anna Lembke unpacks that concept like this:

> With repeated exposure to the same or similar pleasure stimulus, the initial deviation to the side of pleasure gets weaker and shorter and the after response to the side of pain gets stronger and longer, a process called neuroadaptation. That is, with repetition, our gremlins get bigger, faster, and more numerous, and we need more of our drug of choice to get the same effect.[2]

In other words, the more we use something to make us feel good, the more we need it and the less positive return we receive. Before you know it, the good gift, like the food that God gave us to relieve hunger pangs, has become the thing we serve. We have been mastered by dopamine, a pleasure god, rather than the God of pleasure. This is idolatry.

> "Everything is permissible for me," but not everything is beneficial. "Everything is permissible for me," but I will not be mastered by anything.
> 1 CORINTHIANS 6:12, BSB

Sugar is quick and convenient, waiting for anyone in a grocery store checkout line who needs a little pick-me-up of pleasure. Given the constant stress most people live with these days, it's easy to see how people who ignore their feelings and whose minds lack love and optimistic thinking will fall prey to the "quickies" for pain relief.

I'm not saying we need to avoid all sugar, which would be nearly impossible. That's because all food can eventually be converted into glucose, the simplest form of sugar and the energy source your body needs to keep you alive and able to think.[3] Sugar is not necessarily the enemy. It's the overuse and overabundance of added sugars and processed foods (foods with long shelf life) that hurt our bodies and negatively affect our brains.

Sugar is not the enemy. It's the overuse and overabundance of added sugars and processed foods that hurt our bodies and negatively affect our brains.

The Internal Wildfire of Inflammation

For instance, too much sugar can cause chronic inflammation in the body and neuroinflammation in the brain,[4] making it challenging to feel well and think clearly.[5] Like a stress response, inflammation is initially a body's good reaction to a not-so-great situation. When you cut your finger or sprain your ankle, inflammation causes swelling, and swelling isn't always bad. The redness and excess fluid are due to the abundance of white blood cells coming to your aid. Like bodyguards for your immune system, white blood cells hold posts around the infected or injured area to protect it from foreign invaders while healing takes place. Inflammation comes, but with healing and time, inflammation should go.

When we ingest too much sugar, we allow chronic inflammation that fuels the fire of pain inside. When we eat more sugar than our bodies and brains need to function, we turn the fire of our metabolism from a controlled burn, like a furnace, into a forest fire, leaving us to wonder why we don't feel good as the inflammation ravages parts of our bodies.

Chronic inflammation can cause

- joint pain
- bloating
- digestive issues
- skin disorders like psoriasis and eczema
- fatty liver

- heart disease
- high blood pressure
- kidney damage
- sexual impotence
- poor sleep
- weight gain

Too much sugar can also cause neuroinflammation, with symptoms like

- brain fog
- mood and energy swings
- anxiety
- depression
- lack of memory and attention
- behavior consistent with attention deficit disorder or attention deficit/hyperactivity disorder

According to the American Health Association, the average female body needs around 24 grams (or six teaspoons) of sugar a day. The average male needs about 36 grams (nine teaspoons) of sugar daily. Currently, the average American consumes 88 grams of sugar a day (twenty-two teaspoons).[6] That's over three times the amount that a woman needs and just over twice as much as a man needs. Why do we take more than we need? There are many explanations, but I'm convinced one reason is that we don't believe God will provide for our needs, leading us to seek relief on our own.

It's not a new problem. When God freed His people, the Hebrews, from bondage in Egypt, they wandered through the wilderness with few resources. So the Lord provided food from heaven known as manna: "It was white like coriander seed and tasted like wafers made with honey" (Exodus 16:31, NIV). God allocated one omer (about half a gallon) for each person each day, six days a week. They were to eat their portion the day they collected it and not store any for the next day (except for the Sabbath). Some people didn't listen to God. They secretly collected more to ensure they would have leftovers, and guess what? The food spoiled. It stank and was filled with worms (Exodus 16:19-20).

> "Behold, I am about to rain bread from heaven for you, and the
> people shall go out and gather a day's portion every day, that I
> may test them, whether they will walk in my law or not." . . . But
> they did not listen to Moses. Some left part of it till the morning,
> and it bred worms and stank.
>
> EXODUS 16:4, 20

Now why did some people do that? It seems they were concerned that God might not come through the next day, so just in case they manufactured a plan B. They are not so different from those of us now, immersed in a world of endless options and excess, who take in more than we need (or restrict ourselves to less than what we need) because we don't trust God to care for our needs.

Our body-brain, heart-mind, and soul-Spirit connection requires that we live, think, feel, and choose for something greater than either a bag of M&M's or stringent caloric restriction. We are to live believing God will provide for our needs.

When we feel grumpy, tired, and drained, it's a challenge to remain connected to ourselves, much less a God who is Spirit, not flesh. So how can we help ourselves when we're tempted to seek quick comfort for our flesh rather than the God of pleasure who will meet all our needs? One way is to remember these three words from John 4:24: "God is Spirit."

Our Breath: The Fire Extinguisher

At the same time every year, someone presents you with a sweet surprise. A birthday treat! On top, candles blaze as your friends and family sing to you. One secret to taking dominion over your stress is found in this annual ritual. It's not in the cake itself but in what you do just before someone begins slicing it. You close your eyes, take a deep breath, fill your lungs, expand your belly, purse your lips, and blow!

Likewise, whenever you face a test, trial, or temptation, a quick and practical way to lower your stress response and allow the executive region of your brain to override the limbic (emotional) part is to breathe. Not the kind of breathing you do without thinking, but the kind of breaths you take purposefully. Inhaling and exhaling slowly and deeply can ease your stress response. Slow and deep exhales activate your parasympathetic nervous system, which enables your body to "rest and digest" and your mind to gain perspective. In other words, when you take deep breaths, you move your feet back into the stirrups and pull gently on the reins. Another way to imagine the power of taking a deep breath is to picture a broom knocking down the oversensitive smoke detector of the amygdala, which keeps shouting at us to fight or take flight.

When you feel overwhelmed by a negative emotion like anxiety, nervousness, or fear, your sympathetic nervous system can feel stuck in overdrive (fight or flight), and your body will eventually pay with sickness or disease. Focusing on breathing is a quick, accessible, and easy way to keep your body from going into physical and emotional debt.

Focusing on breathing is a quick, accessible, and easy way to keep your body from going into physical and emotional debt.

When adverse moments come, you need the ability to drop into your heart to feel what you feel and to observe what you are thinking. When mad, bad, scared, or sad feelings show up without your invitation, you need to be able to step back and know what you feel and think so you can get to the high tower of your mind—the place of reason, love, and optimistic thinking. Something as simple as taking a deep breath can help you find your way back to the Holy Spirit's leading: "The mind governed by the flesh is death, but the mind governed by the Spirit is life and peace" (Romans 8:6, NIV).

The Greek word for *Spirit* in Romans 8:6 is *pneuma*. The word can mean "wind," "breath," or "spirit," but it is frequently used in the New Testament with specific reference to the Holy Spirit (i.e., the third person of the triune God). It is God's Spirit who animates our lives and enables us to choose in accordance with God's will. We can remember the Spirit's role in connecting us to the presence of God as we move air through our nostrils, which makes it possible for us to move out in the world, thinking and feeling as His children.

In the beginning, God's Spirit kissed our flesh with His breath. He breathed into Adam's nostrils, and His family began. His breath is your breath. He is with you, for you, and as near as your breath. So when you face a moment of distress about the number on the scale or the reflection in the mirror, take a purposeful breath and call on your Father in heaven, asking Him for a greater sense of His presence and peace. His Spirit brings us freedom (2 Corinthians 3:17) and reminds us that we are God's children (Romans 8:15-16).

As you breathe, you take in the oxygen that enters your blood. This is important because some studies show that low blood oxygen can contribute to chronic pain.[7] Deep breathing also helps reduce inflammation; slows the heart rate; increases oxygen in the bloodstream; releases endorphins, which combat feelings of pain; and improves detoxification, immunity, and digestion.

I bet you didn't see this coming. You may have bought this book thinking, *God is going to help me whip this body into shape!* Now here I am telling you to do something as simple as breathing. I'm sure that sounds silly, but the Kingdom of God is counterintuitive to the things of this world. In this Kingdom, small things are big, the last are first, the way up is down, and things that appear foolish are wise.

Citizens of heaven with bodies on earth aren't to try harder. Instead, as therapist Aundi Kolber writes, they try softer.[8] And that looks a lot like remembering to breathe. After all, the breath of God gave you life and now sustains your life. So in moments of temptation, don't freak out. Remember to remain with Him and breathe.

For the Spirit of God has made me,
and the breath of the Almighty gives me life.

JOB 33:4, NLT

You know all those things you keep doing even though you don't want to? All those knee-jerk fight, flight, or freeze responses can be interrupted. Neuroscientist Jill Bolte Taylor describes our ability to regulate our emotions as "the ninety-second rule":

When a person has a reaction to something in their environment, there's a 90 second chemical process that happens in the body; after that, any remaining emotional response is just the person choosing to stay in that emotional loop. Something happens in the external world and chemicals are flushed through your body which puts it on full alert. For those chemicals to totally flush out of the body it takes less than 90 seconds. This means that for 90 seconds you can watch the process happening, you can feel it happening, and then you can watch it go away.[9]

I would retitle the ninety-second rule as the nine breaths rule. You and I have a new way out of old circumstances, and it takes only ninety seconds, or nine breaths, to get there. In fewer than nine deep inhales and exhales, which take approximately ninety seconds, you can move from the valley floor of pain to the high tower of your prefrontal cortex, the place where you can access loving logic and reasoning. When you forget to breathe deeply and purposely for those ninety seconds, you choose to be a coconspirator with your pain. When you remember to breathe purposefully, you give the Holy Spirit a fighting chance to keep you free by remembering the One who gives you breath. He is in charge and wants to help you overcome all things.

Let's hold a fire drill right now so you can practice putting out a fire with your breath.

Sitting down or standing up, place one or two hands on your belly.
  Let your belly fill with air like a balloon.
Inhale deeply, for the count of five.
Exhale deeply, for the count of five.
Call to mind something or even someone that inflames you.
Close your eyes, and breathe the following prayer:
  Inhale deeply, "God."
  Exhale deeply, "I need you."

Sense the presence of God drawing near to you.
Continue this breathing prayer until you gain some peace and
  perspective.

Now you're on the mountaintop in the high tower with your King.

Metabolize

Mind

1. Do you show any signs of chronic inflammation (see page 108) that may be due to your high intake of sugar and/or processed foods?
2. Think of a time you know your actions pleased God's heart. How did that experience compare to the pleasure you get from tasty food?
3. As you learn to focus on your breathing and let God have access to your pain, how might your health and the choices you make be positively affected by these practices?

Mouth

God, Your Word says that You have given me love, power, and a sound mind (2 Timothy 1:7), yet in my moments of pain I look for pleasure apart from You. Teach me how to discover the pleasures of life that are found in You. Holy Spirit, when I am seeking comfort in things more than

in God, arrest me with Your breath. Remind me to breathe. Then take me
to the high place of reason where I am seated with the King. Amen.

Move

God created us as multidimensional beings, so our physical well-being is tied to our emotional, mental, and spiritual well-being. When seeking to address any type of pain, therefore, it is helpful to take the following two steps.

Lower Your Sugar Intake

Although I am not a fan of counting and measuring things as a lifestyle, there's value in taking inventory of what we consume because we can't change what we are not aware of.

Without fear, judgment, or condemnation, and with the gentle guidance of the Holy Spirit who leads you into truth, track how much sugar you eat in an average day.

Instead of being critical of yourself, be curious as a child would be. Before eating something sweet, read the label to see how much sugar it contains. If it doesn't have a label, you can always Google the item. Aim to reduce your intake by one-third per week until you are close to 24 grams per day if you are a woman or 36 grams per day if you are a man. Please remember, legalism should never be your goal. Those are not hard-and-fast numbers. Depending on your activity level, you may need more or less. You simply want to avoid consuming an overabundance of sugar.

Just as with any addictive substance, don't be surprised if you experience a few withdrawal symptoms like anxiety, irritability, or dysphoria (not feeling like yourself). Withdrawal symptoms can tempt you into thinking—wrongly—that feeling bad can't be good and something's not right. Be sure to pray before jumping ship and going back to old ways of thinking, feeling, and choosing. Stay hydrated and remember to practice your deep breathing. When it becomes difficult, use a breathing prayer like the one on page 113. The craving will pass, and each day you don't give in to the pleasures of your flesh, the craving will weaken, and your mind and body will continue to heal.

Breathe

The older you get, the fewer breaths you need per minute. A healthy respiratory rate for an average adult is twelve to twenty breaths per minute, yet many people in today's stressed-out world breathe twenty-five-plus times a minute. Take some time to try the breathing exercises on page 113. Then begin looking for times in your day to connect back to your breath. (I find going to the restroom is a perfect time. After all, it is the *rest*room.)

Combining these two skills of lowering your sugar intake and focused breathing will help you cool your body and brain when your heart and soul feels inflamed by pain.

Meditate

Take ten minutes to listen to the Be Still and Be Loved meditation that goes along with what you just read: https://www.revelationwellness.org/tbr/still/. Then sometime after, lace up your shoes and go for a walk while listening to this link: https://www.revelationwellness.org/tbr/move/.

CHAPTER 11

KINDNESS AND
SELF-COMPASSION

IF YOU HAVE TRIED IMPROVING YOUR physical health but come up short, allow me to ask you this question: Was your desire for change motivated by kindness? Or were shame, frustration, and fear the reasons behind your efforts? If you looked in the mirror and felt disgusted by what you saw, did you try giving yourself a pep talk into doing better and then purge the pantry and the fridge of all tempting foods? And were you surprised—and crushed—when you slipped up?

If so, I have good news and (what may sound at first like) bad news. First the good: I believe God hurts when we don't give Him our hurts and desires, so He offers us a way to come back to Him. The apostle Paul lays this out in Romans 2, where he admonished believers in Christ who passed judgment on unbelievers. These passionate Christians judged those who didn't follow God, but they also stumbled and fell short of God's glory by doing things they didn't want to do. Anyone else guilty of this? Yeah. Me too.

But notice the good news tucked near the end of what at first sounds like bad news:

> Do you suppose, O man—you who judge those who practice
> such things and yet do them yourself—that you will escape
> the judgment of God? Or do you presume on the riches of
> his kindness and forbearance and patience, not knowing that
> God's kindness is meant to lead you to repentance?
>
> ROMANS 2:3-4, ESV

People tend to bristle at the word *repentance*. Every one of us likes to think we are living well as we go about our way, minding our own business. Nobody likes to consider the wrong we are doing or the wrong direction we are going, particularly when it seems as if nobody gets hurt as a result. Repentance gets a bad rap when in fact this gift from God is available to anyone who will receive it. Repentance occurs when we freely choose to turn away from a life without God and toward a new way of life with Him. When we repent, we walk away from selfishness, a life in which we are the center of everything, and we step into a life where we recognize that God is God and we are not.

A repentant person lifts Jesus over the desires that burn within them. They choose to die to their desires and follow God's ways of thinking, feeling, and choosing. John the Baptist prepared the way for Jesus by preaching a baptism of repentance for the forgiveness of sins. John spent his days dunking people in the murky waters of the Jordan River when they came to confess their sins and be baptized—a physical display of repentance, of going a new way. These people were ready for something radically new: Jesus, the Lamb of God who would take away the sins of the world.

If you consider yourself a Christ follower, it's because you had a repentant moment when you put your faith in Jesus, accepting the sacrifice He made when He took your punishment at the Cross. Just like the Prodigal Son, who found himself in a mud pit eating pig pods before returning to his father, so it was for you. The Spirit of repentance pursued you so you could come back to God. "[Do you not know that] God's kindness is meant to lead you to repentance?" (Romans 2:4). It's the kindness of God that makes it possible for you and me to repent and come to Him for new life. For believers in Jesus, new life begins with kindness, and new life is sustained by kindness. It's not the cruelty or even the tolerance of God that leads to our repentance; His kindness makes our new life possible!

What may sound like bad news—our need for repentance—actually gives us access to new life through a new purpose along with new ways of thinking, feeling, and choosing. We are now God's representatives who increase good by sharing the Good News that Jesus saves.

If we try any new thing in our new life in Christ that is not based in kindness, it's not from God and will be difficult to sustain. So as you seek to improve the health of your body, mind, and spirit, pay attention to the way you respond to yourself when you come up short. If the root cause of a thought or feeling doesn't reflect the way God sees you, it may initially lead to behavior modification but will never result in Christlike transformation. Disgust, disappointment, and shame are wildly powerful tools for kick-starting you into change, but they do not have the staying power to sustain change. Only God's love can do that. And God's love is patient and kind (1 Corinthians 13:4).

Disgust, disappointment, and shame are wildly powerful tools for kick-starting you into change, but they do not have the staying power to sustain change. Only God's love can do that.

The Father Who Approves of You

Mary's father is a competitive athlete, known for running the Comrade Marathon in South Africa. (This annual event is the distance of two marathons plus a few extra miles for good measure.) When Mary did well in high school track, her father lavished her with attention—plenty of fist bumps, high-fives, and sweaty hugs. Mary's heart soared when she was in her father's embrace and heard his kind words. Her desire to please him and the self-worth she gained from a win or improved time kept Mary running, even on the days she didn't feel like it. Her brain became programmed to connect performance with acceptance, love, and favor.

As an adult, Mary kept running. One day soon after she'd become a mother, Mary's father made a thoughtless comment about the need for her to do better in her next race to keep from losing her edge. Mary had recently started taking me with her on her runs via my podcast. She was renewing her mind in God's Word while finding new purpose for her life and her body, but her father's comments sent her into a tailspin. While attacking a hill during a training run for an upcoming big race, she kept hearing a voice in her head saying, *You have to push!* The voice became louder and bossier until Mary broke. She couldn't run and cry at the same time. Gasping for breath, she stopped running and started sobbing. Then breakthrough came. She sensed the voice of her heavenly Father saying something very different: *Mary, you don't have to run this hard. I am at the top of this hill waiting for you. I am so proud of you no matter how long it takes you to get up this hill.* Mary says everything changed on the hill that day. God took away her desire to push and strive, replacing it with His loving-kindness.

God's love is patient and kind. It changes the way we view obstacles or approach hills. Striving isn't sustainable, but moving forward in kindness is. Kindness is sustainable because the God who is loving-kindness, who has no beginning and no end, is with us to help whenever we are in need.

When we are hurting, what we need first and foremost is the knowledge that we are not alone and that a presence of loving-kindness is near. This wasn't the norm in my life, and I suspect it was not for you either. In my family, I couldn't go to my parents with hurts because they hadn't healed from their own pain. So whenever I brought them my pain, they were triggered. When my smoke alarm was blaring "FIRE!" my mom and dad did the only thing they knew to do; they fought and fled, leaving me alone and in need.

Nothing in our survival brain is attracted to pain. That is why the love of Jesus is so attractive to those of us in need. He's the friend who sticks closer than a brother (Proverbs 18:24) and the One who will never abandon us in a time of need (Hebrews 13:5).

God doesn't use His Word to "should" on us. God isn't a Father who worries about His reputation, shouting at His kids that they "should" know better and do better or "should" be kind and behave. Giving and receiving kindness isn't something a Christian should do only because it's polite or gives God a good name. While leaving others with a good opinion of our Father is a valid reason to be kind, it's not the most significant one. With loving-kindness, God made us, and we live best with a kind disposition and outlook. Like a supplement, kindness supports our bodies and brains and helps us live well and free. Kindness has been connected to a host of positive effects including longevity, increased energy and pleasure, decreased depression, and a decrease in the experience of pain.[1] Like a mother who pulls her crying baby close to feed, kindness nourishes our whole being. When we are hurting and in pain, God's kindness is sweet.

Like a supplement, kindness supports our bodies and brains and helps us live well and free.

In *The Compassionate Mind*, psychologist Paul Gilbert writes more about the positive effects of kindness:

Children (and adults) who receive kindness, gentleness, warmth and compassion are, compared with those who don't, more confident and secure, happier and less vulnerable to mental and physical health problems; they are also more caring and respectful to others. Receiving kindness, gentleness, warmth and compassion tells the brain that the world is safe and other people are helpful rather than harmful. Receiving kindness, gentleness, warmth, and compassion improves our immune system and reduces the levels of stress hormones. Receiving kindness, gentleness, warmth, and compassion helps us to feel soothed and settled and is conducive to good sleep. Kindness, gentleness, warmth and compassion are like basic vitamins for our minds.[2]

We are hard on others because we are hard on ourselves. We are hard on ourselves because someone we needed to be soft, kind, and compassionate in our moments of pain wasn't. In our hurt we feel exposed and alone. If we sense that no one will be coming to our aid, our emotional survival brain kicks in, and we reach for any sort of fig leaf to cover and comfort us in our helplessness and pain. Over time we come to believe that kindness, gentleness, and compassion aren't very helpful weaponry when trying to survive a world that feels like war.

Empathy and the Mind of Christ

When experiencing hard or hurtful moments, we need to draw close to a person with empathy, someone who is able to be with us in our pain even if they haven't personally lived our experience. Sympathy is not the same as empathy. Sympathy says, "I am sorry you are hurting." Empathy says, "I am sorry you hurt, and I will be with you in it." Sympathy maintains a safe distance while empathy draws recklessly near to those who are hurting and in need.

You've likely felt empathy when someone you love suddenly lost someone they loved. You wanted to do anything you could to be close to them in their grief, but it may have been difficult if you realized that dropping off a casserole seemed to be your only option. How comforting to know that there is nothing we live through that Jesus hasn't also experienced: "For we do not have a high priest who is unable to empathize with our weaknesses, but we have one who has been tempted in every way, just as we are—yet he did not sin" (Hebrews 4:15, NIV). God's empathy and His ability to *be* with you in your suffering is long, wide, and deep.

There is nothing we live through that
Jesus hasn't also experienced.

To process your pain, you need the mind of Christ. It enables you to remain compassionate and kind toward yourself and others who are hurting. Developing such empathy happens little by little. When faced with another's pain, empathy looks for loving and kind ways to meet the need rather than panicking and running away or looking for a fight. When you are willing to remain in the presence of suffering—choosing to take a breath and settle yourself in God's presence—you will be transformed.

So how do you develop empathy? According to nursing scholar Theresa Wiseman, the four actions needed to develop empathy are taking perspective, withholding judgment, recognizing emotion, and communicating emotion:[3]

- You keep perspective when you breathe and stay in the high tower, the reasoning part of your brain, refusing to be seduced by the pain that keeps you stuck in your limbic survival brain.

- You withhold judgment when you remember you are a sinner saved by grace, and the kindness of God saved you. Now, through the embodiment of your faith, others can receive God's kindness too.

- When you think, feel, and choose from a higher perspective rather than from the valley floor, you can recognize your emotions and communicate your needs without having to "do" your feelings through fight, flight, or freeze.

Sin separates, but kindness brings people together. Without kindness, your heart, mind, soul, and body lack integration, and you become like the people Paul admonished in Romans 2—people who confessed their faith in God but had a hard time living it out or loving others. These people heard God's Word and understood that He was kind but never gave their whole selves over to His kindness. Their emotions still held them captive.

Your heavenly Father is kind, and your Father is King. If what you think, feel, and choose is not kind, it's not from Him.

Metabolize

Mind

1. Make a list of the ways God has been kind to you.
2. In the past, what have you done to change your body that hasn't been kind?
3. How does knowing that you have access to God and His kindness change the way you will approach your health?

Mouth

Jesus, You know how hard life has been for me. You know both the unkind things that have been done to me and the unkind things I have done to others. Still You love and pursue me. I need Your mind of empathy so I can treat myself and those who have hurt me with kindness. Fill my body and mind with comfort and kindness when I hurt to keep me from running to the places I've usually gone that don't lead to a life of lasting change. Amen.

Move

Giving and receiving kindness leads to measurable positive effects on the body. When your brain perceives a kind moment, your body releases oxytocin, also known as the love hormone. Oxytocin releases nitric oxide in the bloodstream, which expands the blood vessels, making more space for your blood to flow and lowering your blood pressure. In a moment of kindness, your blood pressure goes down and the strength of your immune system—your ability to fight off sickness and disease—goes up.[4]

If you want to improve your physical health in lasting ways, it's crucial to think, feel, and choose kind things. This is not a selfish act, but a selfless one. You can't give what you don't have. When you receive kindness, you can give kindness.

Before you read on, please take a moment to listen to this short biblical meditation on kindness that I made especially for you: https://www .revelationwellness.org/tbr/still/. If kindness seems as foreign to you as vacationing on the moon, you need this kind of training more than taking a walk, going for a run, or doing push-ups and burpees.

CHAPTER 12

MINDFULNESS AND MINDFUL MOVEMENT

WHILE SHAKING MY TAIL FEATHER with suburban moms in a strip mall aerobics class, I didn't think much about anything, other than how to keep up with the instructor and not look like a fool. That's one of the best things about organized fitness: It's a great way to escape what we can't control and control what we can—like whittling down our waistlines or pumping up our biceps. Mix these feelings of empowerment with exercise-induced hormones, such as endorphins and adrenaline, and you have the perfect cocktail for stress relief.

The problem with using exercise in this way is how fleeting that reprieve can be. Stress comes and stress goes, and so do the benefits of stress relief. At some point, the exercise high wears off, and though our muscles may be stronger and our waistlines thinner, emotionally we're right back where we started. Frustration, anger, sadness, and disappointment can't be shaken off like sweat from our brow. These negatively charged feelings are experienced in our bodies: The related hormones simmer and stew in our tissues while the pathway of thoughts and beliefs in our brains becomes distorted. Negative energy—generated by the way we think, feel, and choose regarding these issues in our tissues—needs to be released or our immune system will be suppressed and our souls depressed. We will feel separated from God's love.

In the last chapter, we learned about four attributes of empathy: perspective taking, freeing ourselves from judgment, recognizing emotion, and communicating emotion. Now let's look at the fifth attribute of empathy: mindfulness. God does not live outside the current moment or rush to judgment; therefore, we don't want to live that way either. Instead, we want to be mindful, filling our minds with the things of God.

Picture someone who lives in survival mode because they are constantly judging themselves and others. Such a person is easily scared and feels out of control when someone or something goes wrong. They do everything possible to get life back under control and make sense again.

Contrast that person with someone who is mindful and can remain calm, regardless of their circumstances. Mindfulness is an awareness, without judgment, of what you are thinking and feeling in the present moment. Take a moment to imagine what your life would look like if you could be present to a challenging moment without getting swept up by the four warhorses of your emotions. Imagine feeling sad without doing sad by bingeing or restricting or jumping to conclusions and saying something you will later regret. Imagine being a person who doesn't rush to judgment but is compassionate and curious. Imagine remaining calm, even in difficult circumstances.

And just to be clear: Using pleasure, apathy, or a guarded heart to numb oneself is not the same as being calm. Calm is an attentive and active state, enabling you to think and feel while remaining in control of what you say and do. Calm is strength under control. The Bible calls it meekness, which is a character trait of Jesus.

> He was oppressed, and he was afflicted,
> yet he opened not his mouth;
> like a lamb that is led to the slaughter,
> and like a sheep that before its shearers is silent,
> so he opened not his mouth.
>
> ISAIAH 53:7

Jesus surely would have preferred to avoid the pain He had to endure on the Cross, but in meekness and a state of calm, He went to Calvary. Jesus didn't yell at the people driving nails into His hands or lose it with the disciples who couldn't stay awake and watch as He prayed in the garden of Gethsemane. Instead, He rested in God's peace. Peace is not the absence of conflict, tension, or discomfort but an awareness that the Father is always near. Jesus could stay calm because He was mindful: His mind was full of His Father's thoughts and words. No wonder, then, that Jesus felt the greatest agony when He was separated from His Father's love: "My God, my God, why have you abandoned me?" (Matthew 27:46, NLT).

The reality is that, because the Father temporarily turned His back on His Son as Jesus took the punishment we deserved, we never have to worry that God will leave us. His grace is particularly evident when we are at our lowest:

> The LORD is near to the brokenhearted
> and saves the crushed in spirit.
> PSALM 34:18

We can put the pain that negatively affects our bodies and our brains to good use, and according to psychiatrist Bessel van der Kolk, author of *The Body Keeps the Score*, mindfulness is key:

> Knowing *what* we feel is the first step to knowing *why* we
> feel that way. If we are aware of the constant changes in our
> inner and outer environment, we can mobilize to manage
> them. But we can't do this unless our watchtower, the
> MPFC [medial prefrontal cortex], learns to observe what is
> going on inside us. This is why mindfulness practice, which
> strengthens the MPFC, is a cornerstone of recovery from
> trauma.[1]

We can't change what we aren't aware of. And to be aware, we must be mindful.

Productive but Not Present

Although technology is a blessing, offering humans an abundance of information, too many people overuse it. The average person touches their smartphone 2,617 times a day.[2] No wonder we are quickly losing our ability to do nothing—to be in and observe our present moment. When's the last time you sat in silence for any length of time without feeling the need to reach for some technology device?

Our minds were designed to experience wonder as we take in God and the world around us. Slowly and subtly, technology has trained our brains and nervous systems to be "productive" every moment. Thanks to technology, there's always a task we can complete while sitting at a red light or while in the carpool pickup line. And if we're not busy finishing a task, we can always fill the void of stillness with entertaining distractions like Netflix or another scroll down social media lane (even when we were just there fifteen minutes ago). When's the last time you stood in line at the grocery store, and rather than looking at your phone, you noticed the people around you? Or when was the last time you took a walk without your phone? A brain on an abundance of busy is a brain that resists silence and stillness and views quiet as something to avoid and run from.

Technology has trained our brains and nervous systems to be "productive" every moment.

A person stuck in a busy brain habit loop may find it difficult to process their pain since they aren't aware of how they feel or what they think. As a result, they are quick to react and judge. In addition, living with a brain stuck in busy mode contributes to chronic stress, which negatively affects the way our brain operates, overloads our nervous system, and suppresses our immune system, making us more susceptible to sickness and disease. Round and round on the hamster wheel we go all day long until we collapse into bed at night. Sleep is good for us, but rest is available not just when we sleep but during our waking hours. We can find rest when we push away from distractions to be still and know (Psalm 46:10)—to be mindful of God.

Keep in mind that awareness is intertwined with mindfulness. Our lives were not made for unceasing duty or distraction but for delight in God. The Lord wants aspects of His Kingdom to come to earth through us, but to be His agents, we must be willing to be interrupted—even when the alarms, texts, and email notifications from this world have distracted us. God wants to break through our busyness to give us more of Himself and His peace.

So how do we stay mindful of His peace? We look to Him:

You will keep in perfect peace
all who trust in you,
all whose thoughts are fixed on you!
ISAIAH 26:3, NLT

Two Ways to Cultivate Mindfulness

1. Mindfulness through biblical meditation

Biblical meditation is a powerful way to practice peace.

Before you freak out because I used the word *meditation*, allow me to put your mind at ease. We're not talking about the kind of meditation in which you tuck your legs into the shape of a pretzel, sit on a rubber mat, light some incense, and chant gibberish. We aren't trying to empty our minds and think of nothing (good luck with that anyway). For the Christian, meditation isn't emptying our mind but filling it with the thoughts of God. We do this best when we get still and simply be.

---

*For the Christian, meditation isn't emptying our
mind but filling it with the thoughts of God. We
do this best when we get still and simply be.*

To be clear, studying Scripture is not the same thing as meditating on Scripture. When we study the Bible, we are seeking knowledge, understanding, and wisdom about God and His ways. Studying is for students who want to learn. With the help of the Holy Spirit, we seek to understand the significance of a passage in the context of which it was written, along with its meaning for us today. Studying God's Word informs us about God. It's good to hunger to know more about God. But just like eating food, it's possible to choke on our food if we don't chew it.

In fact, to avoid choking, aid in digestion, and obtain the most nutrients, experts have long advised people to chew food at least thirty-two times before swallowing it.[3] When we meditate on Scripture, we put the meat of God's Word into our mind and chew, chew, chew. Anyone can bite into and know something about God's Word, but I suggest that it's in chewing, thinking about, and keeping His Word on our mind that we are nourished. As we meditate on Scripture, we roll the words of God over and over in our mind, withdrawing nourishment from them. God even promises that, as we meditate on His Word, things will go well for us—and that includes in our bodies and brains:

> This Book of the Law shall not depart from your mouth, but you
> shall meditate on it day and night, so that you may be careful to
> do according to all that is written in it. For then you will make
> your way prosperous, and then you will have good success.
> JOSHUA 1:8

What can it look like to "chew" on the Word of God? The first thing to do is read it. You need to eat! Open your Bible and pray for the Holy Spirit to sit down and eat with you. Read God's Word until a particular verse or words from a passage grab your heart. Now begin to chew. Take a few belly breaths, soften your body in your chair, and read the words repeatedly. Do not strive as you repeat the words.

Your goal isn't to memorize Scripture, but to give the Word time to speak to you personally. Just like a mindful eater is aware of the different flavors and textures of what they are eating, a person practicing biblical meditation allows the different flavors and textures of God's Word to come to life. We might taste the sweetness of God's comfort or the bitterness of conviction regarding a circumstance in our life. If conviction comes, don't let your meditation time end before you receive the presence of God's comfort. As you close your meditation time, pray and ask the Holy Spirit to bring this Scripture to mind as you go about your day. And finally, look for opportunities to savor that Word again, such as when you're walking across the parking lot into the grocery store with a cart full of kids, as you brush your teeth before you go to bed, or as you're in your office cubicle and sense your body start to stress.

Biblical meditation is a means of giving ourselves permission to wonder at God's goodness. Just as we marvel when we look at the stars, so we are awestruck when we pay attention to God. Observant people are less condemning and more curious, as well as less frustrated and more fascinated, by other people and things. Instead of popping off in a moment of pain, observant people are less likely to take offense and cling to hurt.

Biblical meditation is a means of giving ourselves
permission to wonder at God's goodness.

---

2. Mindfulness through self-awareness

The Prodigal Son demonstrates the power of being honest about his own situation: "When he came to himself, he said, 'How many of my father's hired servants have more than enough bread, but I perish here with hunger!'" (Luke 15:17).

This wayward son, who'd left his father's home in search of something more, had wasted his inheritance. Only now, while covered in mud and eating pods meant for the pigs, he finally "came to himself" or "came to his senses" (NIV). The son was mindful, which gave him perspective (the first attribute of empathy). He didn't stay buried under the weight of his rebellion and sin but put thoughts of his father's goodness at the forefront (prefrontal cortex) of his mind. He knew he needed help and who might give it to him.

When we meditate, we are being mindful. Mindfulness strengthens our mind's ability to observe, come to ourselves, feel what we are feeling, know what we are thinking, and see ourselves or others without judgment or condemnation.

Coming to ourselves is a grace given to us by God. It enables us to observe ourselves being tempted by our emotions so that, rather than giving in to rebellious ways, we can go to Him with our needs. I used to be taken captive by every emotion that came my way. That ended years ago when my relationship with God totally changed. I had prayed over and over that the Lord would keep my children from the same trial I experienced growing up. When it happened anyway, I was devastated. In all honestly, when this bad news hit, I was red-hot angry at the Lord. I felt completely let down, forgotten, and betrayed by Him. Here I was, a ministry leader who'd given her life entirely to God, yet He had allowed something terrible to happen to me and my children. My heart was tired from yet another heartache. For a brief moment in my fatigue, I considered being done with this living for Jesus thing. In deep pain, I had absolutely no desire to open my Bible and read.

One morning, exhausted and disoriented by the pain, I wandered into my study. I flopped my body down on my corduroy couch—the place I would regularly meet with God. Flummoxed and fatigued, I just sat there and stared at the wall. I told the Lord I was mad at Him and wouldn't open my Bible. As I sat there, I sensed these words in my spirit: *Good. Stop studying and come to Me.*

> You search the Scriptures because you think that in them you
> have eternal life; and it is they that bear witness about me, yet you
> refuse to come to me that you may have life.
> JOHN 5:39-40

I had the same heart condition as the Pharisees. In John 5:39-40 Jesus rebukes them for being so busy studying and enforcing the Scriptures that they had overlooked the essential thing: Him! Despite all their knowledge about God, they'd missed the main point of studying the Scriptures: intimacy with God.

Reading and studying His Word is necessary so that disciples can learn about God and follow where the Holy Spirit leads. We can then go, proclaim, and teach. But sitting and meditating on Scripture is for the children of God who simply want a hug from their Father.

Those of us who live in a first-world country with religious rights and instant access to the Bible through numerous websites and apps do not perish because we don't have access to His Word. I suggest we perish because we lack intimacy with the God of the Word. We don't need more information about God but intimacy with God. To transform anything, including our pain, we must read and meditate on the Word of God, learning to come to Him like children and to simply be. It's good practice to be still and know (Psalm 46:10) before we go and do.

It's good practice to be still and know
(Psalm 46:10) before we go and do.

Mindfulness as Self-Care—and Health Care

Mindful meditation doesn't just reap spiritual benefits but physical ones as well. In 2011 psychologists at Harvard University studied the effects of mindful meditation on the brain. They scanned the brains of the participants before and after mindfulness meditation training. After eight weeks of instruction, the researchers discovered positive structural changes in the parts of the brain responsible for controlling stress and improving memory, attention, sense of self, and empathy.[4] A 2017 meta-analysis (a summary of many studies on the same subject) found that participants who incorporated mindfulness meditation in their weight-loss protocol were more effective at improving their eating behaviors and losing weight.[5] And another 2017 meta-analysis study found that people who meditate have lower levels of the stress hormone cortisol and other physiological indicators of stress.[6] High cortisol levels can contribute to higher amounts of abdominal fat. Researchers at the University of

California, San Francisco, found that when a group of overweight women practiced mindfulness and mindful eating, not only did their anxiety and markers for chronic stress decrease but . . . get this . . . so did their belly fat.[7]

Practicing stillness and meditation have also been shown to reduce anxiety, age-related memory loss, blood pressure, and pain; improve emotional health, attention span, and sleep; control pain; and help fight addiction.[8]

People who meditate are literally brain architects. As they might redesign their house, they are remodeling their brain through meditation, which has been shown to decrease the size and activity of the amygdala (smoke detectors for danger) and increase the activity of the medial prefrontal cortex (high towers). This means that people who meditate are less reactive to life and more responsive to people in need, including themselves. Instead of taking flight, going to fight, or freezing because of perceived danger, mindful people can step back to observe what's going on and choose not to react with panic and pain. They keep their agency. They keep perspective. They feel what they need to feel without falling into a pit of despair. They remember that they are the beloved of God who belong to Him and can talk to Him about their hurts and needs. He brings the gift of His peace, in addition to offering them His love, presence, and empathy: "Peace I leave with you" (John 14:27).

Being mindful doesn't have to be limited to the times you are purposefully quiet and still. Be mindful when you move. Mindful movement is what we are doing together when I direct you to a link and invite you to move with me. Exercise (movement) not only strengthens your bones, lungs, and muscles; more importantly, for the purposes of this book, it improves your brain health through the release of neurotransmitters and hormones like dopamine, serotonin, norepinephrine, and acetylcholine. These chemicals create a positive effect on your mood and lower depression and anxiety. And people who exercise increase the size of their hippocampus, an area located in the limbic brain that is responsible for learning, long-term memory, and mood.

The hippocampus is one of two places in the brain where neurogenesis, or the creation of new brain cells, occurs. Neurogenesis is necessary for neuroplasticity, the reorganizing and restructuring of the brain toward improved

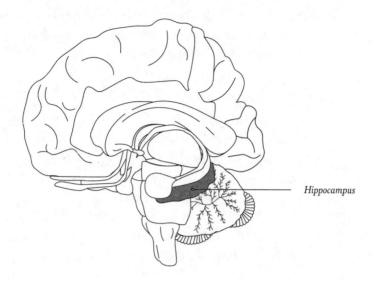

Hippocampus

health.[9] In essence, moving our bodies improves our cognitive ability to remember, learn, and think. So doesn't it make sense that when we move our bodies and think about the Word of God and His presence with and love for us, we not only strengthen our bodies but our brains, improving our ability to learn, memorize, reorganize, and operate in line with what God says is true and best? Little by little, day after day, as we replace unnecessary busyness with stillness and move through our day mindfully with God, we become new.

Meditational movement increases oxygen and blood flow to your brain and allows you to engage with God without the protective act of judgment or the denial of emotions connected to painful memories. So don't be surprised if a well of emotion suddenly comes over you and you begin crying as you move. As I like to say, this is just God moving the issues out of your tissues and softening you with love.

Metabolize

Mind

1. How attached are you to busyness? How comfortable are you with being still? Why?
2. Do you study and/or meditate on God's Word? How does each feel to you?

3. How could the practice of being still or engaging in mindful movement be helpful for you? What are some specific ways this could improve your body's health?

Mouth

God, I want to be a student of Your Word. I want to be Your child who can come to myself to come to You. Give me a hunger to study Your Word more than a hunger for the things of this world. Help me use my knife and fork to cut into the meat that is Your Word. Then help me remember to chew, chew, chew what I eat. Help me to slow down, be mindful of Your nearness every moment, and take time to chew the food I eat—whether food for my body or the daily bread of Your Word that nourishes my soul. Heal my body and brain as I choose to slow down, be Yours, and move out into the world in love. Amen.

Move

If you don't already have a habit of meditational stillness or movement, don't feel like you have to devote hours to start. Ten minutes a day for stillness and twenty minutes a day of mindful movement will do.

Take ten minutes to listen to this Be Still and Be Loved meditation, which goes along with what you've just read: https://www.revelationwellness.org/tbr/still/. Then sometime before you read the next chapter, lace up your shoes and go for a walk while listening to this link: https://www.revelation wellness.org/tbr/move/.

Humbling Yourself

I will arise and go to my father, and I will say to him, "Father,
I have sinned against heaven and before you. I am no
longer worthy to be called your son. Treat me as one of your
hired servants." And he arose and came to his father. But
while he was still a long way off, his father saw him and felt
compassion, and ran and embraced him and kissed him.

LUKE 15:18-20

CHAPTER 13

HUMILITY, NOT HUMILIATION

Simon and I were married in fall 1997. By the fall of 1998, it looked as if we wouldn't make it past one year. I had fallen into the same desire trap that my mom had. I needed a man to love me. One dark and stormy night, the words "I don't think I can be married to you anymore" rolled off my husband's tongue. I was devastated.

Within hours, I was driving through the desert, back home to my parents' house in Arizona. While buckets of rain fell from the sky, hot tears filled my swollen eyes. *I can't believe I'm about to be divorced* and *What's wrong with me?* looped over and over in my head. I knew it was time. I needed God. The seed my coworker had planted just a few months prior when she invited me to church was starting to bloom. All my body-sculpting, clean eating, and other attempts to look good on the outside couldn't seem to fix my insides. That night everything changed for me. On the heels of this bad news, good news was on the way. Like the Prodigal Son, I was ready to come home to God. I brought my whole body, with all its pain and my muddy heart, so I could return home to Him. While there was still a long road to travel on the journey to healing and wholeness in my marriage, the first stop on my road trip was home—home to God.

When we find ourselves in a painful mud-pit moment, God's grace makes it possible for us to come to ourselves, which I define as the ability to step outside ourselves so we can see who we are and what we've done without feeling condemned. At the same time, it enables us to be mindful of the choices we've made and take personal responsibility for them. The question is: What will we do with the knowledge that something is wrong with us and we need to change?

> *God's grace makes it possible for us to come to ourselves:*
> *to step outside ourselves so we can see who we are*
> *and what we've done without feeling condemned.*

Years ago when Oprah Winfrey was in the thick of her weight-loss efforts, I watched her interview a woman who'd written a book about food and God. The author talked about God in a spiritual way but not according to the tenets of a specific faith. Oprah hung on every word this woman said and began to connect the dots of her physical desires with her spirituality.

Oprah had one of her classic aha moments (which is another way of saying a "coming to yourself" moment). She connected the adversity she'd experienced growing up with her ongoing struggle to lose weight. Oprah emphatically affirmed the author's message by sharing the pep talk she'd given herself the night before. She said something like, "I told myself, *Oprah, we are no longer that little girl. We are a big girl now. Those painful days are behind us. We can let those things go and get on with our life. We don't have to deal with our pain this way anymore.*" The audience erupted in thunderous applause. On the surface, just deciding to grow up and behave better sounds like a good plan. But I remember feeling confused as I watched, thinking, *Oprah, I don't think that's going to work. Things don't go away just because we tell them to. But Jesus, the God you are all talking about without* really *talking about, came to offer a remedy for our pain.* Not only did

Christ come to take the penalty of our sin upon Himself; He came to be our advocate: "Therefore he is able to save completely those who come to God through him, because he always lives to intercede for them" (Hebrews 7:25, NIV).

Jesus put on flesh, faced the same temptations as we do, suffered, and overcame death and the grave; as a result, He has the power and authority to help us in our time of need. We need only to yield our pain to Him. We don't need to pull ourselves up by the bootstraps, grow up, and suck it up. We need to lower ourselves in godly humility, which *Easton's Bible Dictionary* defines as "a prominent Christian grace. A state of mind well pleasing to God that preserves the soul in tranquility and makes us patient under trials."[1]

Worldly humility focuses on the self and can lead to humiliation if you can't seem to do the things you know you should do or stop the things you know you should stop doing. For example, you tell others you're getting healthier by starting a new diet and investing in a personal trainer, only to be right back where you started months later, maybe with a few extra pounds to boot. Trying to change into a better version of yourself can be downright frustrating and self-condemning when change is determined by you and is completely riding on you. It's too much responsibility for any one person to bear, no matter how much knowledge or power, or how many resources, you have.

Exercising Humility

With an Irish father, an Italian mother, and three siblings, Tracy grew up in a home that never lacked emotional energy. Tracy's father was a hard-working blue-collar man who ended his day with at least a six-pack of beer. Her mother's behavior was erratic and unpredictable; late in life, she was diagnosed with bipolar and obsessive compulsive disorder. Then at age thirteen, Tracy was sexually abused by a family member.

Tracy found a way to escape the unpredictability and trauma by becoming a three-sport high school athlete, only to be sexually abused again at age seventeen by an athletic trainer who'd been hired to help her get a college sports scholarship.

A few years before, at age fifteen, Tracy had given her life to Jesus after being invited to church by a friend. She welcomed Christ into her heart but had no understanding of how to release her pain to Him.

In college she met a wonderful guy who became her husband. Years later, now married, and with a family of her own, she found that her unprocessed pain was surfacing in discontent. As an escape from her pain, Tracy engaged in every sporting endeavor she could find—running, mountain biking, long-distance triathlons—anything to keep herself from noticing the feelings hiding just under the surface of her skin. Looking for further relief, Tracy turned for comfort to another woman in her sporting community. For two years they had a secret affair, even though both were married. Eventually, wracked with guilt, Tracy couldn't take the weight of her shame. Tracy "came to herself" when she knew the only way to be released from the weight of her guilt was to come clean. Surrendering the outcome to God, knowing she could lose everything, she confessed her wrongdoings to her husband. By God's grace, her husband was willing to stay with her, and they began an intense time of therapy. But overwhelmed with the effort of trying to process all her feelings of shame, guilt, and humiliation, Tracy turned to alcohol.

Knowing that Tracy liked to run, her therapist recommended that she start listening to the *Revelation Wellness* podcast as she exercised. During her next run, Tracy was wrecked—moved to tears—as she listened. In His fierce love for her, God was accessing the deep issues that were stored up in her tissues. As she moved her body, the truth of God's love for and acceptance of her started to click. The revelation that God has been with her, is not ashamed of her, and gives her the power to overcome her temptation to seek relief apart from Him is helping and healing Tracy more and more each day.

Tracy's story is an example of godly humility. Without her love for God and her desire to be clean, she would still be running from Him and relying on other things to cope with her pain. Godly humility is preserving her soul and her family, while also increasing her strength and tranquility.

Pride is the opposite character trait of humility. Pride grows in our hearts when we make things about us. For those who grew up in a home where it felt as if nobody was there to take care of them, pride develops as a survival tactic, making it hard for a self-reliant person to ask for help when in need. Tracy had emotional needs that weren't being met, and she had learned to lean on herself rather than God. Whether physically, financially, mentally, emotionally, or socially, learning to lean on God first and most for everything helps us stay in good health and grow in godly humility.

---

*Learning to lean on God first and most for everything
helps us stay in good health and grow in godly humility.*

Trying to improve any area of our lives (work, marriage, family, money, or physical well-being) without the input and guidance of the God who made us is like trying to construct a house without blueprints. Christian author Elisabeth Elliot once said, "We cannot give our hearts to God and keep our bodies for ourselves."[2] Yes, and amen! We are to submit our whole selves, including our bodies, to God in view of His mercy. God is the creator, sustainer, and redeemer of all things. Real transformation begins and is sustained through ongoing godly humility.

This humility comes from God, not ourselves, and it leads us to repentance; a desire to do life in a new way with new purpose. In godly humility, we relinquish control of our lives and the meaning we've given our pain. Humility helps us take our right place in the order of creation. We bow our lives to a King while surrendering the weapons we tried using to manage our pain. We give God the right to repurpose our pain and to tell us who we are as His people. We know that, no matter what trouble comes our way, we must give Him the right to lead us because He showed us the Way when He won back our lives in one great act of humility.

Have this mind among yourselves, which is yours in Christ Jesus, who, though he was in the form of God, did not count equality with God a thing to be grasped, but emptied himself, by taking the form of a servant, being born in the likeness of men. And being found in human form, he humbled himself by becoming obedient to the point of death, even death on a cross. Therefore

God has highly exalted him and bestowed on him the name that
is above very name, so that at the name of Jesus every knee should
bow, in heaven and on earth, and under the earth.

PHILIPPIANS 2:5-10

One major factor that will keep us stuck in a cycle of pain is holding on
to the things we think we are owed because of the bad hand we were dealt.
When life doesn't go the way it should have, we grasp on to our pain like a
security blanket or, even worse, make it part of our identity. A "hurt person"
will often cling to their hurt identity, thinking they have permission to hold
everyone and everything hostage.

Some people who've been hurt take another route. They draw on God's
common grace—the ability to recognize their survival tendencies and dis-
cern how pain has negatively affected their body-brain connection—so
that they learn how to express their feelings constructively and develop
good coping skills. The truth is, just about everyone can dust themselves
off after a failed attempt, rise from their mess, clean up, and try a new
approach. A good self-help strategy is part of common grace. Don't get
me wrong, I love a good personal development course. I love to be challenged, to grow in knowledge and change. *But* when it comes to my heart,
its longings, and its proclivity toward deception, I need to know God first
and most.

Rather than following my heart, I need to follow Jesus'. Rejected by
His own people, spat upon, scorned, and shamed, Christ didn't cling to
His rights as God. He humbled Himself to the point of death on the Cross
so you and I could transform and transcend our pain (Philippians 2:6-8).
We can be reconciled back to God and take back our purpose, subdue and
have dominion, and restore our stolen identity.

So far we've moved through the first stage of understanding the pull
of our desires and how misplaced desires create pain, and in the second
stage how pain negatively affects our bodies and brains. Now in this
third stage we begin the amazing work of transforming our pain through
godly humility. It's at this point that everything changes, but only for
those who do not consider their bodies their own and are willing to lay
down their whole selves for Christ's sake. Our ability to come to ourselves

and turn toward God is godly humility, which is not a common grace given to everyone. Instead, it's an amazing grace for people called by God that keeps them from living with body shame and minds that can be deceived.

Humbling ourselves takes us into higher reasoning. Humbling ourselves gives us access to God's Kingdom, His world of inside-out, "nothing is impossible," transformational change.

Putting Humility at the Heart of Decision-Making

Want to know if you are following Christ with godly humility? Ask yourself these two questions whenever you feel stressed-out and lacking peace.

1. Is what I am thinking, feeling, and choosing to do kind?
2. Will what I am stressed out about matter in a thousand years?

Is what I am thinking, feeling, and choosing to do kind?

As we learned in chapter 11, God's *kindness*—not His anger or impatience—made a way for us to repent and live with a higher purpose. If what we are thinking, feeling, and choosing isn't kind, we can be sure it's not of God and lacks the humility that leads to new ways of doing life. Kindness is not compulsive but thoughtful. It is reflected by a get-to, not a have-to, mentality.

Compulsion says, "I have to eat more fruits and vegetables. I'm unhealthy, and the doctor told me so."
Kindness says, "I get to eat more fruits and vegetables. Consuming foods that lower inflammation in my body would be kinder for my body and my brain."

Compulsion says, "I have to forgive. God said so."
Kindness says, "I get to give away the grace I've received from God. When I choose to forgive, I will set both of us free."

A humble person wants more God at all costs. More God means more kindness.

Will this matter in a thousand years?

Asking yourself this question in a moment of tension is a kind and wonderful way to stay humble and hold your peace with a heavenly mindset. In Christ, you are a new creation. You are a citizen of heaven. Heaven is your home. Your Kingdom life started the day you put your faith in Christ. You now live from heaven to earth, submitted to a good and all-powerful King. That may make you might think, *Great! Then who cares about my body? It's temporal and not going with me to heaven.* But you are forgetting two crucial things:

1. King Jesus' desire is to bring more of heaven to earth, and your physicality is how you make His Kingdom seen. If you think, feel, and choose to do things that conflict with that heavenly mindset, your body will feel at war with your mind. You might confess your faith in God with your tongue, but how you live out your life, in your body, will look and feel contrary to your belief.

2. The apostle Paul tells us we have citizenship in heaven, from where Christ will return and "transform our lowly body to be like his glorious body" (Philippians 3:21). So, yes, our body is an eternal concern to our eternal God. One day we will have a body in heaven. As we live out our lives in our earthbound body, we must remain aware of what our heart desires and the actions of our body. *Will this matter in a thousand years?* If what our body wants will positively affect our character and ability to become more Christlike, we can bet the answer is yes! Everything that doesn't contribute to that needs to fall away.

By the way, in moments of stress, we often lose our ability to step back and observe our hearts. Asking these two questions requires us to be mindful. That is one important reason that a stillness meditation appears at the end of each chapter. Please don't skip them.

Living a new life with God—the life we were designed to live in the Garden of Eden—was never meant to be done in our own ability. We need God's help. We live and experience life because we have bodies. These bodies, which enable us to experience life, are meant to be our heavenly dwelling places on earth. Ongoing humility and bowing our hearts and desires to God are the keys to accessing the safety and transformed lives we have with Him. If we stay humble, submitting our pain and desire to God, we will never again lose the key to our body-home.

Metabolize

Mind

1. Jesus says, "Those who exalt themselves will be humbled, and those who humble themselves will be exalted" (Luke 14:11, NIV). What does this verse mean to you?
2. Think of a concern you have about your body. Then answer these two questions:

   Is what you are thinking, feeling, and choosing kind? If the answer is no, what could you do to change it into something kind?

   Will this matter in a thousand years? Think more eternally. How does God want to humble you to see the matter of your body from a higher and heavenly place?

Mouth

God, I need a new way to think, feel, and choose when it comes to my body and the pain it holds. I lay myself and my pain before You. Thank You for Your amazing grace, which makes a way for me to come to myself so I can come to You. You gave Yourself completely for me, so now I give myself completely over to You. You can have my heart and my body. In light of eternity, I ask You to heal my mind and the way it is connected to my body. Amen.

Move

Take ten minutes to listen to this Be Still and Be Loved meditation: https:// www.revelationwellness.org/tbr/still/. Then sometime today, lace up your shoes and move for twenty minutes while listening to this link: https:// www.revelationwellness.org/tbr/move/.

CHAPTER 14

HELP!
A FOUR-LETTER WORD

When I gave birth to our first child, Jack, any pipe dream or expectation I carried around in my heart about motherhood went up in smoke. If trauma can be defined as anytime life doesn't go the way we think it should, leaving us feeling as if we're unable to cope, becoming a mom for the first time was definitely traumatic for me.

Jack had colic. And when I say *colic*, I'm not speaking of the kind when a baby is fussy for a couple of hours a day. Oh no. Jack screamed bloody murder, day and night, night and day, for ten weeks straight. Jack's cries were not just due to a few gas bubbles stuck in his belly. Jack's cries came from intense pain, which caused him to lose weight. I felt as if I were failing as a mother, unable to help my son thrive. Eventually, Jack was diagnosed with a list of food allergies and extreme reflux. In short, his digestive tract was not well. Beyond our switching him to a crazy-expensive formula and administering reflux medicine daily, only time would bring him relief. For ten weeks, I got only thirty to forty-five minutes of sleep at a time. My body brewed in a hormonal-sludge stew, and parts of me leaked, cracked, and bled. I felt like I was surviving a war or living someone else's bad dream.

Growing up, I'd always found a way through complex circumstances. The challenging environment I grew up in had made me very resourceful. If something needed to get done to make things better, I would figure out a way to do it. In this situation with my son, however, I could do little more than wait. But waiting and watching my son in physical pain triggered my own pain. I cried out to God all the time, especially since I spent so little time sleeping. And although I knew God was there for me, it often felt like He wasn't. I needed His help, and I needed help from someone wearing skin.

Then one day I heard a knock at my door. As soon as I opened it, my new friends from church came flooding in as if on a military rescue mission. One woman made a beeline for the kitchen and assumed her post at the sink. Another commandeered the laundry basket, swooping up baby socks, crib sheets, and Simon's workout clothes, all of which had been lying in the corner for a week. Melinda, the captain of this mommy-saving brigade, grabbed me by my shoulders. Then she firmly pinned my arms to my sides, walked me to my bedroom, and said, "You are going to lie down now, and you're going to get some sleep. We are here to help." I burst into tears. I'd been found out. I didn't have it all together. As Melinda pulled back the sheets and I lay down, a feeling of relief swept over me.

People who live through hard things often have difficulty asking for help. Once upon a time when they needed help, nobody came. The last thing they want to do is ask for help. Since the people who were supposed to be there for them didn't come through, they don't want to risk having the same experience again. So these people get resourceful. Finding a way to endure suffering is not just nice but necessary. For some people, the gallon of ice cream in the freezer or the cookies in the pantry will do; others will turn to the drugs and alcohol their friends are using.

Learned helplessness is a term coined by the American psychologist Martin Seligman to describe what happens to someone when they feel trapped in an adverse environment. He used a classical conditioning study with dogs to illustrate what this means. Seligman would ring a bell, which was followed by a shock to a dog. Naturally, that dog would jump back in response to the shock. Ring a bell. Shock the dog. Dog jumps. Repeat.

After a while the dog would respond to the bell ringing as if he had been shocked, even though he hadn't. Bell rings. Dog jumps—even though he hadn't been shocked. Next Seligman put the dogs in a cage. The floor in half of the cage produced an electric shock while the floor on the other side did not. The cage was divided by a low fence so that any dog could see the other side and easily jump over it. The dogs who had previously been shocked were put in the side that produced shocks through the floor. Instead of jumping to the other side, they lay down and accepted the shocks, as if there was nothing they could do to escape. Even after being placed in a new environment where they could escape the shocks, they had been conditioned to believe no help was coming and there was nothing they could do to change their situation. On the other hand, when Seligman put a dog that hadn't been shocked on the electrified side of the cage, the dog instinctively jumped the fence to the other side.[1] This is a great picture of learned helplessness—the belief that we can do nothing to escape our situation.

It's easy to see how learned helplessness works to help a person survive. Consider the child of an alcoholic father or resentful mother who never knows the emotional environment they'll return to after school. Like a shocked dog, they believe their only option is to tolerate the adversity and get through it. The part of their brain that is developing and designed to help them think reasonably and optimistically (the prefrontal cortex) is underactive, while their emotional brain (the amygdala) remains diligent and calls the shots. Young people who feel helpless are prone to view the world through a lens that tells them, *I am alone. Nobody is coming to help me.* That affected my outlook and the choices I made when my mother exposed my father's sin to me.

Learned Helplessness vs. Learned Helpfulness

If you think about it, the term *learned helplessness* is a little misleading. A person doesn't learn helplessness; we are *born* helpless. Depending on our stage of development, there's only so much we can do. Infants wail as a way to communicate their needs. One-year-olds cry because they can't get to the kitchen for a snack when they're hungry. What children need to learn is helpfulness. Our ability to learn helpfulness depends on the people around us and the environment we live in. If you were raised in a relationally healthy home, with parents or guardians who made themselves available to you when you needed something, most likely you learned helpfulness. As your brain was forming, whenever you had a need or felt confused by something, you knew you had an advocate, someone on your side who was safe and could help you. Of course, not every one of our needs is met nor is every question answered. But when most of our needs are responded to, we learn to love and trust others and to become helpful ourselves.

The first thing a hurting person needs is to know they are not alone. The actual resolution of the problem—if fixing it is even possible—is secondary. You've probably seen a war movie in which a soldier is mortally wounded with an injury that no amount of gauze or surgery will fix. But what often happens? A platoon buddy throws down their weapon, rushes to their comrade's side, sweeps them up in their arms, and holds them close to let their dying friend know they are not alone. The war buddy gently rocks their wounded friend while locking eyes with them and saying, "It's okay. I'm here."

Likewise, when you are in pain, ideally another person's caring presence, not a pint of ice cream, will provide comfort. When we're hurting, presence *is* help. When we're in trouble, we want to know we are not alone. The psalmist reminds us that, not only is God our source of power, but He is also right beside us: "God is our refuge and strength, a very present help in trouble" (Psalm 46:1).

Since you picked up this book, it's probably safe to assume you are looking for help with your body and your mental health. You're tired of feeling as if something is broken in your body or as if, when God handed out the workout genes, you didn't get a pair. You just want God to show up and do something, anything, to help get you out of your misery. But friend, if you feel like God has failed you or hasn't helped you in the past, I suggest it's not God or your body that is failing you. Instead, it's where you are looking for help that is faulty and a little off: "No one can lay a foundation other than that which is laid, which is Jesus Christ" (1 Corinthians 3:9).

Security Begins with the Foundation

I love New York City. The sights and sounds. The buzz and energy of people as they hustle about the streets. The views at the top of the iconic Empire State Building, from which you can check out NYC's skyline. You can't pay money, however, to look at the most important part of that building—the foundation. That 102-story Art Deco building, completed in 1931, stands even today because of the solid foundation on which it was built. If its foundation begins to slip or crack, the risk to the people who live or work in it goes up. Architects and civil engineers agree that the taller and more complex a building's design is, the deeper and more complex its foundation must be. In other words, it's what is hidden underground that makes it possible for us to see the beauty above ground.

Jesus doesn't invite us just to believe in Him but to follow Him. And followers of Christ are builders. We don't build alone; we build alongside the Holy Spirit—the one Jesus said He leaves with us as our Helper. Through the Holy Spirit, a new foundation is laid in us, and that foundation is Christ. When we build on Him, our old foundation—a self-reliance built on fractured beliefs and our desires for a pain-free life and flawless body—is slowly but surely taken down. A new foundation for a new life built on Christ alone is laid. He doesn't just help us but saves us, both now and in the future.

Reality check: How often do you go to Google to find answers when you feel fat, ugly, or old? How often do you look for help in your social media feed? Recent surveys tell us that the average person spends about 145 minutes per day (almost two and a half hours) on social media (and that amount of time has increased every year since 2012).[2] How many of them are searching for the "help" they need online, rather than seeking support elsewhere? Now how often do you go to God to ask for what you need *and* give Him time to provide it? You will know you've gone to Him with your needs because after doing so, you will have His peace.

> Don't worry about anything; instead, pray about everything. Tell God what you need, and thank him for all he has done. Then

you will experience God's peace, which exceeds anything we can understand. His peace will guard your hearts and minds as you live in Christ Jesus.

PHILIPPIANS 4:6-7, NLT

Notice that it's not just in asking that we receive God's peace, but it's asking with thankfulness. In gratitude we remember who God is and all that He's already done for us. Thankfulness activates the MPFC, the high place in our brain where reasoning takes place.

Next time your pants feel tight and you're tempted to respond with disgust, take a moment to breathe. Taking an intentional breath slows down the emotional commotion occurring in your limbic brain. An intentional breath can become your prayer for God to come and help you find something to be thankful for—like the fact that your legs are strong and able to get you where you need to go or the fact that you are alive to hug someone. We never hear someone on their deathbed say, "I wish I had lost more weight."

I'm not suggesting that being thankful and going to God in prayer and asking for help is easy, particularly when so many other quick-and-easy resources are vying for our time and attention. But don't forget, the salvation Christ provides is your foundation. And that foundation is strengthened and built as you go to Him in prayer with thankfulness and ask for His help.

Salvation is not the result of a one-time request for help. Not only did Jesus deliver you from darkness into light, from death to eternal life, but He will save you from wasting an hour or two scrolling online or spending money on a quick fix to relieve your pain. Don't stop asking for His help.

The Life-Giving Help Found in Hope

In the 1950s Curt Richter, a psychobiologist and professor at Johns Hopkins University, did a series of experiments on rats. He put them in buckets filled with water to see how long they could swim. Even though they are known for being good swimmers, the rats lasted only minutes before they drowned. In a follow-up experiment, he pulled the rats to safety just before they went under. After giving them a short period of rest, he put the rats back in the buckets. This time, the rats swam another sixty hours or so! Takeaway: Help doesn't just give us a reprieve from our pain; it gives us hope to keep going.[3]

Help doesn't just give us a reprieve from our pain; it gives us hope to keep going.

When the mommy-saving brigade invaded my home that day, they did more than finish my laundry and allow me to get some sleep. They didn't just give me help; they gave me hope. And hope is like a supernatural, heaven-sent power pill for a weary soul, body, or mind. Jack's colic was not going to stop in one day. It was going to take time. I needed hope—the strength to keep going, to lean into a future time when Jack wouldn't be in constant pain and crying day and night. And so it is for you. Even as you draw on God's strength and help, improving your health will not happen overnight. It will take time. The first changes will be hard to track and see. You can't measure healing that starts in the deep and hidden places of your past pain. Eventually healing will make its way to the outside, but as you wait, keep asking for help. Receive hope by remembering and being thankful that Jesus saved you, is saving you, and will continue to save you. He will not let you sink. Remember, He saves! Persevering through suffering produces hope:

> Not only that, but we rejoice in our sufferings, knowing that
> suffering produces endurance, and endurance produces character,
> and character produces hope, and hope does not put us to shame,
> because God's love has been poured into our hearts through
> the Holy Spirit who has been given to us.
> ROMANS 5:3-5

Before following Christ, we were like those swimming rats with the capacity to last only minutes before heading to the bottom of the bucket. We were helpless and without hope. We were stuck, chasing after temporary pleasures and vanity in an effort to ease our hurts and fears. We thought perhaps another round of calorie control or bingeing would do. Before Christ, we were totally helpless, feeling stuck with the bodies that hold our pain. We were eternally separated from God, caught in a cycle of sin and misplaced desires, which took a toll on our physical body and brain. We were utterly helpless and headed for ruin. We needed help of the highest kind.

Two of my favorite words in the Bible are "But God."

> But God, being rich in mercy, because of the great love with which he loved us, even when we were dead in our trespasses, made us alive together with Christ—by grace you have been saved.
>
> EPHESIANS 2:4-5

God sees your weakness, your feeling of "stuckness" when it comes to your body and the way you relate to food, family, and friendship. He knows how others have let you down and didn't help you when you needed it most. But He is not that kind of Father or friend. Every time you humble yourself and turn to Him for help, the Holy Spirit takes a sledgehammer to your old foundation—your "get through and stay safe" mentality. Your faith in Jesus Christ is the solid foundation on which to build your health, body, finances, and relationships.

Knowing you need help isn't a sign of weakness; it's essential for more of God's power to get in. Asking for help does not mean you are a failure; it means you are building your foundation of faith. Asking for help in everyday life is required for those seeking hope for their future.

Knowing you need help isn't a sign of weakness;
it's essential for more of God's power to get in.

Because God is so rich in mercy, He offers us grace, and it's by this grace that we are saved. Grace means we can't do anything to earn God's love or help. Calorie counting and clean eating won't solve our feelings of helplessness. God was helpful when we were helpless. He is our ever-present help. He is always near. And although our circumstances won't often change overnight, He can use these troubles to restore what we have lost. We can subdue and take dominion, be fruitful and multiply, and live according to His image in us, which was His idea from the beginning: "Let us make man in our image, after our likeness" (Genesis 1:26).

Let Him help you use your circumstances to transform you so that you become more like Him.

Metabolize

Mind

1. Think of a difficulty you've experienced sometime in the last few years. How easy has it been for you to ask for help?
2. What negative emotions (mad, bad, sad, or scared), feelings (expressions of those emotions), and felt sense in your body (tight, constricted, tingly, fluttery) show up when you reach out for help?
3. When it comes to your health, where do you see learned helplessness affecting your thoughts and behaviors?
4. Based on what you've read in this chapter, what do you think God wants you to know about the help He provides?

Mouth

God, my Father, I come to You now asking for Your help because You know everything about me. You know the circumstances I've lived through that cause me to think and feel helpless. You know how this pain erases the peace You give and want my body to hold on to. I no longer want to merely survive and make it through another day. I want a new life. Be my foundation for everything I think, feel, and choose. When I turn to other ways to cope because I'm tempted to believe I am alone and no one is coming to help, remind me that You are with me. You are my ever-present help. Amen.

Move

Take ten minutes to listen to this Be Still and Be Loved meditation: https://www.revelationwellness.org/tbr/still/. Sometime today, lace up your shoes and move for twenty minutes while listening to https://www.revelation wellness.org/tbr/move/.

CHAPTER 15

KEEP GOING;
IT'S ONLY A TEST

When my marriage was in the pits, I humbly came to the Lord. But I came alone. Simon was fine with me attending church; he just had no interest in going with me. My husband comes from a line of British agnostics with a keep-calm-and-carry-on spirit. Yet as Simon watched me change as I got closer to God, he became curious. One night as we were sharing a plate of tiramisu, Simon asked if he could go to church with me. As those words hung in the air, my heart fluttered and my soul silently squealed. After weeks of investigating and researching like the good engineer he is, Simon became a believer.

I don't have the word count to go into all the details, but within a few months, Simon was questioning and backpedaling out of the Christian faith. Eventually he declared himself an atheist. I was all in on following God and living out His purposes for my life. And I was married to an atheist who didn't hesitate to verbalize his distaste for the church and his belief that I was being deceived. Oh, the pain. I was so mad at God. I felt set up and sucker punched. Why would a God who supposedly loves me answer my prayer that my husband would love Him as I did, only to let the enemy take Simon away? Nothing about this felt like the actions of a good God.

I share this part of my story because I've observed that many people who decide to follow God wholeheartedly find that life gets more challenging once they do. Maybe, like me and the Prodigal Son, you came to your senses and in humility asked God for His help. You were saved. But being saved hasn't led to the eradication of your pain. Perhaps life has gotten harder and feels even worse. All your believing and praying don't seem to be working, and God's help feels more like an idea than a reality. After a short honeymoon period with the Lord, we discover that we still live in a broken world with an enemy who wants to destroy us. This reality hits us hard and brings more pain.

Now that we are in the workout phase of this book, let's not let this rattle us. Just as twenty minutes into a workout session when you feel the burn in your hamstrings or labor to breathe, you know you are hard in your pursuit of God as you feel resistance from your enemy. When you are moving toward godly change, things tend to feel harder before they get better. The heat is on!

Yet we can feel our feelings without doing our feelings. We may feel like quitting, but that doesn't mean we quit. We can persevere because we have the grace of God on our side and the presence of His Holy Spirit in us. As we humble ourselves before God and ask for His help, Satan, the enemy of God's goodness, is stirred up. He is opposed to you knowing and loving God because he knows that when you do, there's no stopping the goodness you can give to others. Satan is done for when the men and women of God are willing to let the Lord have it all—their hearts, minds, thoughts, emotions, and bodies. Through our lives, we can make the beauty of God's Kingdom—an unseen reality—visible.

Satan doesn't care who or what we worship, or who or what we give our time and attention to—as long as it isn't God. While our heavenly Father is jealous *for* us, Satan is jealous *of* us. The present ruler of this world once had intimacy with God, the One who created him and knows him best. Satan lost this treasure when his obsession with his own beauty made him proud and led him astray:

You were blameless in your ways
from the day you were created
till wickedness was found in you.
Through your widespread trade
you were filled with violence,
and you sinned.
So I drove you in disgrace from the mount of God,
and I expelled you, guardian cherub,
from among the fiery stones.
Your heart became proud
on account of your beauty,
and you corrupted your wisdom
because of your splendor.
So I threw you to the earth.

EZEKIEL 28:15-17, NIV

While our heavenly Father is jealous
for us, Satan is jealous of us.

Not only does Satan oppose us and feel jealousy toward us, he's also predictable. He is actually quite boring; after all, God is the source of creation and creativity, not him. All Satan can do is take what God has made and called good and twist it with his lies for the purpose of producing more and more pain on the earth. Satan is a one-trick pony show. His ploy? Keep the image bearers of God focused on the stuff that looks wrong or is going wrong with themselves, others, and the world. Keep them living on the valley floor of pain. Satan loves to make life hard for the blessed people of God. He knows people with hard lives are more likely to harden their hearts toward the kindness of God. If Satan can keep us away from God's love, he can keep us from repentance; the ability to course correct and go a new way with God. Doing life God's way enrages our enemy.

One Step Forward, Another Back

Meghan grew up a pastor's kid and considered herself a good Christian. At every age—young child, preteen, teenager, and young adult—she attended all the church events one person could endure. She witnessed her father's pleasure when she did all the right Christian things and his silent treatment when she fell short. Meghan had a major falling out with her dad when she fell in love with a boy in her youth group and things went a little too far. Meghan became pregnant at age seventeen, and this small-town scandal almost wiped out her father's call to ministry along with an entire church. Shamed and shunned from her community, Meghan kept her baby—and the pain of rejection. That hurt went with her into single motherhood.

Meghan moved away from home as soon as she could. Burdened by shame and the ongoing stress of providing for her young daughter, she tried to soothe herself with food late at night. She eventually realized that her overeating would be harmful long-term for both her and her daughter, so Megan reached out to Revelation Wellness for one-on-one online coaching with me. "When it felt like everyone was turning their backs on me, food became my closest friend," Meghan told me early on.

With God's help and my guidance, Meghan started making strides in the right direction in just a few weeks. The connection between her mind and body was beginning to "click." Her energy was up, her eyes were bright, and she felt empowered to make healthier decisions for herself and her daughter. One day after a time of movement and mediation, she rose from her mat with tears in her eyes and said "Alisa, I've been a believer my whole life. But today I met Jesus." Those words hung in the air. We knew we were standing on holy ground. Meghan was healing—giving God all her attention, her heart, her pain, and her body.

Then one day, trouble came. Her now ten-year-old daughter got sick. Really sick. She was diagnosed with a rare bone disease. Consumed by fears of her daughter suffering and the shame of feeling at fault, Meghan went into a full-blown tailspin. I gently pointed her to a verse from Scripture that illuminates why Christians should not be shocked by the troubles of this life:

Beloved, do not be surprised at the fiery ordeal among you, which
comes upon you for your testing, as though something strange
were happening to you.

1 PETER 4:12, NASB

God is kind and life is hard. It's difficult to reconcile a God of kindness
with the many difficulties we face. But we can't afford to lower our trust in
God and His supreme loving-kindness so we can hang out in the valley of
our pain. God's plan for our lives requires us to persevere—to rise from our
messy mud pits and follow Him so we can grow up. After all, how does a
child grow emotionally, intellectually, and physically? Through testing in
school and life.

In Exodus 3 God came to Moses in the wilderness as he tended his
father-in-law's sheep. In the heat of the day, Moses noticed a burning shrub
that wasn't being consumed. Moses walked closer to get a better look at
something so strange. From out of that bush God's voice told Moses that
he had been chosen to lead his people out of Egyptian captivity and into
the place where the Lord's people could worship him: the Promised Land.

I have surely seen the affliction of my people who are in Egypt
and have heard their cry because of their taskmasters. I know their
sufferings, and I have come down to deliver them out of the hand
of the Egyptians and to bring them up out of that land to a good
and broad land, a land flowing with milk and honey, to the place
of the Canaanites, the Hittites, the Amorites, the Perizzites, the
Hivites, and the Jebusites.

EXODUS 3:7-8

As we work to transform our own pain, we can notice several things in
this interaction between God and Moses:

1. **Moses was aware and alert.** He wasn't distracted by bleating sheep,
   his hunger or thirst, or the heat of the day. He wasn't (metaphorically) looking down at his phone while scrolling through his social
   media feed. Moses noticed the burning bush. Thank God for Moses'

awareness; otherwise, he might have kept walking and missed his call. Sure, God could have set up another time for Moses to meet with him. In fact, who knows? Maybe Moses had already passed by several burning bushes. But remember: Nothing changes without awareness. Awareness occurs if we are mindful, being in the present moment without judgment. Mindfulness is crucial for moving out of captivity and into freedom.

2. **God knows our pain.** God was sending Moses to go on His behalf to secure His people's freedom. He sees the affliction of His people and hears their cries "because of their taskmaster." The Hebrew word translated here as "taskmaster" is *nagas*. This term refers to "oppressing," "driving," "exacting," or "exerting pressure."[1] Satan notices when people move toward prosperity of soul and peace with God. He's quick to press against that. He assigns taskmasters that he hopes will wear us out and harden our hearts with the binding agents of fear and unbelief. Taskmasters are anyone or anything that stresses out God's people! God hears our cries, and at the right time, He will act. While we wait, the tension created by our taskmasters will test us and strengthen us.

3. **Opposition is allowed for our advancement.** Notice that God tells Moses He will free His people from captivity and bring them into "a good and broad land, a land flowing with milk and honey, to the place of the Canaanites, the Hittites, the Amorites, the Perizzites, the Hivites, and the Jebusites." What? God plans to deliver His people from captivity, only to send them to a new home that is controlled by foreign enemies, future taskmasters in waiting? It's true. Just because God delivers His people from captivity doesn't mean we will never have to deal with our enemies again. He works through us to put creation back in proper working order. As God's image bearers and children, we are to subdue and have dominion over those enemies who oppose good so we may worship God and walk in His freedom. Just as testing in school demonstrates that we have what it takes to advance to a higher grade, so God's times of testing prove we know God and through faith in Him we have power to

destroy the plans of the enemy. We've been trained and transformed by the Spirit—the power of God. We've been tested and tried and know how to use the weapon of His power and authority. As we advance God's Kingdom, Satan loses territory.

Four years after her diagnosis, Meghan's daughter is recovering, but Meghan's own health has suffered. She's been diagnosed with an auto-immune disease. Meghan admits she lost herself during those four years and is resolved to start again. For a short time, she tasted freedom in her body and wants it back. Meghan knows her return to wholeness begins with receiving the loving-kindness of God, which means refusing to shame herself for neglecting her body.

After getting together again for our first session, Meghan rose from her mat with tears in her eyes. She said, "Jesus wants me to know that He realizes how hard that time was for me. Although I may have given up on myself, I didn't give up on Him. He's proud of me." Though she had lost herself after her daughter's diagnosis, Meghan hadn't lost sight of God. Because of the trouble she's endured, she loves God and other people more deeply. She is advancing. She is taking back holy ground.

In Christ, You Are Never a Failure

You're more than halfway through our "workout class," which is designed to help you transform your pain into purpose. When life feels hard or appears bad, put no confidence in what you see. Help is on the way! God knows your pain. You're being tested, so don't quit. God doesn't expect you to pass every test with flying colors, but He does expect you to learn from your failures. As a matter of fact, in the New Testament, the word translated *disciple* means "a learner" or "a pupil."[2]

God doesn't expect you to pass every test with flying colors, but He does expect you to learn from your failures.

The Bible calls us to be children of God—not adults of God, business professionals of God, or personal growth experts of God. Children grow through learning, and as we follow Christ throughout life, we will always be learning, taking tests, and sometimes failing.

On the other hand, failing never means you are a failure. When you know you've blown a test, bring this acronym to mind:

F—frequent
A—attempts
I—in
L—learning

If you keep showing up without judging yourself or others so you can continue to learn, you are doing it right!

To live an embodied faith, you must remain mindful, present to the moment without judgment. Keep taking the tests. With God's help, you will break up and break through the pain. You are taking back whole and holy ground.

Take a deep breath in as you count to five; then exhale for a count of five. Now repeat after me: *This is only a test.*

Metabolize

Mind

1. In the past, how have you been tested when you started taking steps to improve your health?
2. How will you respond differently now that you know such tests will surely come?
3. How can you keep from living unaware of Satan's schemes? Why does he not want you to live well and free from your pain?

Mouth

God, You know every trouble that's going to come my way. I know You test me because You want me to know that, with You, I have what it takes to overcome all things. You are teaching me how to access the power

and authority I have in You to take captive all things that threaten the
health of my body and soul. In the name of Jesus, I put all the tricks
and whisperings of Satan under my feet. Help me not to despise times of
testing but to see them as opportunities to become more mindful of You,
to come to You and receive Your power and authority. Help me to advance
in the Kingdom and advance Your Kingdom on earth, as it is in heaven.
Amen.

Move

Take ten minutes to listen to this Be Still and Be Loved meditation, which goes along with what you've just read: https://www.revelationwellness.org /tbr/still/.

Sometime before moving on to the next chapter, lace up your shoes and go for a walk while listening to this: https://www.revelationwellness .org/tbr/move/.

CHAPTER 16

WORKING FROM REST

THE FEW TIMES I'VE CHECKED into a hospital, I've never been asked what size workout shoe I wear or if I would like to see the gym before I put on an open-backed cotton gown and lay down in bed. Treadmills, ellipticals, and dumbbells may be housed in the rehabilitation wing, but when you're admitted to the hospital, your treatment is generally centered in one place: a bed. That's because hospitals are a place for hurting people to go so that others who are physically stronger and medically wiser can care for them. And bed rest is generally a major part of recovery.

In Mark 2, we see Jesus relaxing around a table, eating with sinners and tax collectors. A few scribes and Pharisees are there as well. (I think of these religious types as overworked religious people with hypervigilant amygdalae who live in stage one survival mode, trying to preserve their sense of safety and control under the reign and rule of the Roman empire.) They ask the disciples why their teacher keeps such scruffy company. Overhearing, Jesus replies, "Those who are well have no need of a physician, but those who are sick. I came not to call the righteous, but sinners" (verse 17).

Like the patient who is rushed to the ER or admitted to the intensive care unit, we are all dependent on God's mercy and healing touch. We mean well in our attempts to protect ourselves and others from bad things, but due to the generational effects of sin, we are all sick. And Jesus is our Physician.

Too often, however, we resist His loving care. I suggest that all of us who put our faith in Christ have a hard time aligning our thoughts, feelings, and choices with God's commands. Jesus came for the sick, and we come to Him sick, stuck in survival mode. When we live that way, it's hard to trust our heavenly Father and other people. We think no one has our back, no one loves us, and most certainly no one can do anything as good for us as we can do for ourselves. We believe the lie that we can't let our guard down or take a day off. We must stay vigilant, keeping watch over our own lives.

In all our efforts to stay safe, we forfeit our God-given right to rest and heal. Just as I had to be ambushed by my friends and literally pushed into bed to rest, our overactive amygdalae and overstressed bodies won't take a break until we believe that any help that comes can be trusted. Hurting people find it hard to trust in the positive effects of rest. But just as Jesus trusted His Father as He slept peacefully on a boat during a storm (see Mark 4:35-41), we can trust and rest in our Father too.

This is what the Sovereign LORD, the Holy One of Israel, says:

"In repentance and rest is your salvation,
    in quietness and trust is your strength,
    but you would have none of it."

ISAIAH 30:15, NIV

Many of us struggle to rest; we want to do good but are living through bad times. As with asking for help, allowing time for rest feels shameful and makes us feel as if we are weak. Instead of taking the rest that repentance brings, we choose to "have none of it." We fail to realize that in God's Kingdom all good work begins from repentance and rest. If we want to rebuild our bodies or brains to live in better health, our foundation must be Christ, and the first crossbeam of support we erect for our body-home must be rest. Our ability to get quiet and then still our anxious hearts, working hands, and worried minds in God's presence strengthens our faith.

In fact, rest is the first thing we did with God before we got to the work of subduing and having dominion:

> The heavens and the earth were finished, and all the host of them. And on the seventh day God finished his work that he had done, and he rested on the seventh day from all his work that he had done. So God blessed the seventh day and made it holy, because on it God rested from all his work that he had done in creation.
>
> GENESIS 2:1-3

God created all of heaven, earth, and every bird and sea creature in five days. On the sixth day He made all the land animals and the first two people: man and woman. Then on the seventh day, God rested. It's interesting that even though He blessed us and purposed us to multiply good on the earth, humans' first day on earth was not spent cutting back the begonias or tending sheep. Their only assignment was to spend time resting with Him. God didn't need to take time off, for He has eternal power and strength. But like a good Father who doesn't just tell His kids what to do but shows them how to do it, He modeled the joy and spiritual discipline of rest. He took the whole day off so He could enjoy creation with His kids.

Working from a Place of Rest

That brings us to another point: Children of God don't work *for* rest, they work *from* rest. Just this morning, I heard a successful fitness influencer share on Instagram that she'd recently been diagnosed with an autoimmune disorder. She said it flares up only when she is stressed and overworked, but she confessed that slowing down and resting are not easy for her.

Children of God don't work for *rest; they work* from *rest.*

In the same Instagram story, she mentioned that she'd recently broken an annoying habit. When asked how she did it, she said she did the same thing she'd done to overcome her eating disorder years prior: She got busy on a new project so that she didn't have time to think about the things that fueled her annoying habit. In other words, getting and staying busy—the same thing that caused her illness to flare up—was her solution to breaking a poor habit loop.

I share this illustration not to call her out but to call out the inconsistencies. We're all guilty of cognitive dissonance; holding conflicting values. My point is this: As people of God, if we don't start a new work from a place of rest, that new endeavor won't be fruitful. Without rest, we will continue to transfer our pain from one form of destructive energy to the next. Without rest our immune systems will be overworked and when the first wave of a life-storm hits, we'll be wiped off our feet. Jesus still extends this invitation to you and me: "Come to me, all who labor and are heavy laden, and I will give you rest" (Matthew 11:28). Exhaustion is not a sin. It's a sign for us to investigate our hearts to make sure we are not giving more importance to someone or something other than God. When we are overworked, overstressed, and tired, we can lose perspective on life. We can be quick to forget who we are and what we are living for.

The Old Testament prophet Elijah has much to teach us about exhaustion and losing perspective. In 1 Kings 18, we read how he personally took on the 450 false prophets of Baal in Israel, telling them he could prove they were devoted to a false god—one who could neither hear them nor save them. One man against 450. Imagine the amount of stress Elijah must have felt! Surely his heart beat faster, his palms sweat, and his stomach turned after he made his challenge. After all, Elijah was human. Still, he did not shrink back.

Instead, he watched as the false prophets, despite their wild wailing and antics, could not get Baal to rain down fire to consume the animal they'd sacrificed. When Elijah prayed aloud to God, on the other hand, the Lord sent fire down from heaven to burn the sacrifice Elijah had made to him. The Israelites immediately bowed down to worship the true God, and at Elijah's command, they rounded up the 450 false prophets, who were then slaughtered.

But soon after his Super Bowl–sized halftime moment of faith, Elijah was confronted by a messenger from Jezebel (who along with her husband, King Ahab, had introduced Baal worship in Israel). The courier told Elijah that the queen was seeking revenge and planned to kill him. Elijah ran.

> He himself went a day's journey into the wilderness and came and sat down under a broom tree. And he asked that he might die, saying, "It is enough; now, O LORD, take away my life, for I am no better than my fathers." And he lay down and slept under a broom tree. And behold, an angel touched him and said to him, "Arise and eat." And he looked and behold, there was at his head a cake baked on hot stones and a jar of water. And he ate and drank and lay down again.
>
> 1 KINGS 19:4-6

Notice what Elijah did. He lay down and slept—twice. Elijah was exhausted. This super prophet who believed in the supernatural power of God was not Superman. Like you and me, he was a natural man. He was empowered by the supernatural Spirit of God, yet limited to the constructs of the natural world. His exhaustion had hindered his ability to operate from his high tower and think clearly. In fact, when Elijah first confronted the false prophets, we see hints of that weariness in his declaration that "I, even I only, am left a prophet of the LORD" (1 Kings 18:22). He had fallen prey to the common lie "I am all alone" that often accompanies suffering and fatigue.

Yet even in his weariness, Elijah had shown up before 450 evil men to make God known and seen. Afterward, however, the feeling of being alone was more than he could bear. After facing off with 450 evil men, he was running from one scorned woman.

Having come to the end of his own strength, Elijah was losing perspective. Then God's loving-kindness showed up. He didn't shame His prophet for being weak. Instead, He met Elijah in his limitations by providing the basics that Elijah needed—sleep, food, and drink. Likewise, if we want to be ready to hear and do the will of God and fight our enemies, we must have the basics in order: food and hydration (which we've discussed in previous chapters), as well as sleep and rest.

Sleep vs. Rest

There is a difference between sleep and rest, but both are essential to maintain a robust connection between your body and mind. First, let's talk about sleep.

As humans with physical bodies who live in a limited physical world, we can't avoid our need for sleep. In fact, at some point if we don't get it, our muscles will no longer be able to support our frame, and we'll collapse. If you've ever seen a tired toddler's head bob and weave until their head falls face-first into a plate of food, you've witnessed this uncontrollable phenomenon.

When we sleep, our eyelids close and we become unconscious of the world around us. Just as our smartphones eventually stop working when their operating systems are outdated, the systems of our bodies that keep us upright, consciously thinking, feeling, and choosing throughout our day stop working when we fall asleep. This allows a night crew of other systems to get to work, cleaning up the day's waste and by-products.

Sleep provides the following health benefits:

- Boosts the efficiency of our thought processes, enabling us to make better choices the next day
- Removes toxins from our brains that have built up during waking hours
- Organizes and files new information learned that day
- Solidifies memories
- Leads to more creative and optimistic thinking when challenges occur
- Regulates appetite, which helps prevent excess weight gain
- Reduces stress and strengthens the immune system, both of which are related to a lower risk of chronic illness and disease
- Boosts metabolic system and muscle recovery, especially important for people who regularly exercise
- Improves mood throughout the day[1]

According to the Center for Disease Control and Prevention, an adult requires seven or more hours of sleep per night.[2] But the quality of sleep matters. Getting a minimal amount of sleep will keep us alive, but getting good quality sleep enables us to grow and thrive. Poor sleep disrupts our immune cells, which increases inflammation that contributes to heart disease, obesity, arthritis, diabetes, and cancer as well as our ability to fight off infections like the common cold.[3] When poor sleep continues for an extended period, some people become anxious every night around bedtime, worried they won't get enough sleep.

Rest is not the same as sleep. Sleep is an unconscious state, while rest is a conscious state of being. A person who embraces rest looks for moments in their day to steal away with God. For instance, meditation, which we discussed in chapter 12, can improve quality of sleep at night and help those who struggle with insomnia.[4] Some people shy away from meditation, however, so Andrew Huberman, a medical doctor and neurobiology researcher at Stanford, introduced the term *non-sleep deep rest* (NSDR).[5] I like this term because it explains exactly what it is: deep rest that isn't sleep. And you don't have to sit down on a mat with your eyes closed for thirty minutes to reap some of the benefits of NSDR.

Though Dr. Huberman advocates accessing NSDR through yoga nidra or hypnosis, I believe we can achieve deep rest simply by taking a minute or two to sit or stand before stretching mindfully and breathing deeply. If you are at work and want to be refreshed on a day with multiple meetings, I encourage you to take a few minutes of rest between them. Drink water, look out the window, breathe in and out, pause, and reflect without judgment. At a red light, instead of checking your phone for incoming texts, embrace a moment to sit and be.

Here's a rest challenge for you: The next time you go to the bathroom, don't scroll on your phone or multitask your thoughts. Rest, "take care of business," breathe, and simply be. As I've mentioned before, it is called the *rest*room.

You can become a person of rest, and rest is something you can do during the day. When you feel anxious about something like a critical meeting at work or a phone call you don't want to make, you can turn your sense of restlessness into a cue to take a breather and invite God into the stress. People of rest know they need more of God's presence, not another scoop of ice cream or thinner thighs. People who practice rest during the day are better able to hold their tongues and seek God's face rather than reacting to stress by fighting, taking flight, or freezing.

You can turn your sense of restlessness into a cue to
take a breather and invite God into the stress.

Purposefully look for restful moments to mindfully connect yourself back to God, the source of all life! Now more than ever, in this frenetic, fast-paced, noisy world, we need to practice being people of deep rest. Be sure to prioritize sleep at night and seek moments of rest during the day. As pastor and author Mark Buchanan said, "Unless and until we rest in God, we'll never risk for God."[6]

God's invitation to enter His rest still stands today. Will you take it? I sure hope so.

In the remaining chapters, we will delve deeply into the world of faith, the place of rest from which you do good work and find courage to take the risk of standing against the opinions of the world when necessary.

Who's ready to rest in God and take some risks?

Metabolize

Mind

1. Have the difficult events you've lived through affected your sleep? If so, how?
2. Read 1 Kings 19. How does Elijah's story of fatigue resonate with you?
3. How do you rest during the day, especially in stressful moments? If taking time to rest feels unnatural, ask God what He would like you to do and then record what you sense Him telling you. Try to write as if He were talking directly to you.

Mouth

God, Your Word says You give Your beloved sleep. Thank You that You give me sleep during the night and rest during the day because I believe in You. Help me become a person who does all things from rest and not for rest. Amen.

Move

Notice how many hours of sleep you get per night. Then on a scale of 1 to 10—1 being poor and 10 being excellent—rate the quality and amount of sleep you get.

Consider implementing a sleep routine that includes rituals you do every night before bed. For example, my phone alarm goes off at 8:45 every night, reminding me that it's time to get ready for bed. Before hitting the sack, I set out my vitamins for the morning, prepare the space for my morning quiet time, and place my morning workout clothes in clear view. I then put on my PJs, cleanse and care for my skin, brush, floss my teeth, and slide into bed with no phone. All of this takes about twenty minutes.

The following ideas can also improve the quality of your sleep:

- Shut down electronic devices two hours before bedtime.
- Minimize noise and light in your bedroom. The quieter and darker, the better your sleep will be. Consider getting blackout shades. (I recently got some and absolutely *love* them!)
- Adjust the temperature in the room as needed. Between 60 and 69 degrees is recommended for most people. Start there and adjust according to your needs.

When it comes to rest, you've been practicing NSDR every time you've done a Be Still and Be Loved meditation at the end of a chapter. Keep going! I promise you—and the research backs me up—this practice will heal and strengthen your body-brain connection.

Now begin to look for small windows of time in your day to expand your practice. Next time you're in line at the grocery store, look around and breathe rather than mindlessly scroll on your phone. Get curious about the people around you. When going from one work meeting to the next, take two to five minutes to deliberately rest and breathe. Steal away moments with God, thanking Him for the blessings of that day. These quick moments of rest, along with your focused meditation times, will create more resilience in your body and brain to think, feel, and choose what's best, even in moments of pain.

Finally take ten minutes to listen to this Be Still and Be Loved meditation: https://www.revelationwellness.org/tbr/still/. Then sometime today, lace up your shoes and go for twenty minutes of movement while listening to this link: https://www.revelationwellness.org/tbr/move/.

The
Cooldown

Staying the Course

And the son said to him, "Father, I have sinned against heaven and before you. I am no longer worthy to be called your son." But the father said to his servants, "Bring quickly the best robe, and put it on him, and put a ring on his hand, and shoes on his feet."

LUKE 15:21-22

CHAPTER 17

NO LONGER ORPHANS: YOUR NEW IDENTITY

I HAVE FRIENDS WHO HAVE adopted children born in extreme poverty. It's not uncommon for these children, now living in safe and loving homes, to hoard and hide food. Some of these babies had gone directly from their mother's womb to a street corner, where they were left for dead. After being found by good Samaritans, they were placed in orphanages with too few adults to care for the babies in need. Without someone to provide consistent care in the form of a warm cuddle, a belly tickle, or an adoring gaze, the children's emotional development languished.

It's easy to see why food became a great substitute for comfort and care. If you experienced extreme hunger, think how comforting a belly full of food would feel and how strongly your brain would begin to associate comfort with food (and its accompanying release of dopamine). Food has the power to fill a tangible void through the feeling of a full stomach. It comforts like a hug on the inside since food never talks back, shames, or sends someone to their room. Food satiates physical hunger pangs and meets our emotional need for comfort and security.

But we don't actually have to be orphans to have a skewed relationship with food. It's possible to be born into luxury with worldly power and possessions yet lack love and attachment. For some of us, our home of origin perhaps felt more like an orphanage, a holding place, until the day God adopted us. This is especially true if we were raised in homes where we saw little evidence of God's loving-kindness or were taught "truth" while being pressured to suppress our feelings.

Like the Prodigal Son, we may think the things of this world can fulfill our hearts and quench our need for love, belonging, safety, and control. An orphan spirit may have taken root, leading to a lack of trust in God and difficulty loving ourselves and other people. Orphans may find creative ways to stay alive, but they will never do more than survive until they stop running and turn to God. Fear is the primary source of energy that fuels an orphan spirit, and only the Father's love can chase out all fear.

> For all who are led by the Spirit of God are sons of God. For you
> did not receive the spirit of slavery to fall back into fear, but you
> have received the Spirit of adoption as sons, by whom we cry,
> "Abba! Father!"
>
> ROMANS 8:14-15

God has chosen us, spiritual orphans, not out of pity but delight. He comes to give us a new life without fear, a new identity as His child, and a divine destiny to go and tell others they are invited into our Father's house too.

Knowing we would encounter pain in this life, God entrusted us to our earthly parents until the day we would cry out for His help and so be saved and adopted into His family. In the Father's house, the testimony of the trouble He has delivered us from and the tests we've taken become the rocket fuel for our divine destiny.

The children of God can be secure in their identity: "You are no longer strangers and aliens, but you are fellow citizens with the saints and members of the household of God" (Ephesians 2:19). God, the King of all creation, is our Father, and His refrigerator is always full. We eat because we are hungry, not to fill needs that only God can meet.

With God as our Father, we eat because we are hungry,
not to fill needs that only He can meet.

Membership Has Its Privileges

Welcome to the cooldown phase—the time to enjoy the benefits of all your hard work. This is where the good stuff happens. It's your turn to lie down on your little piece of brown carpet, stare at the ceiling tiles, and sense God's love for you after all the hard work you've been doing (and not just reading about) so far. Don't skip the cooldown! Don't be those people in a group exercise class who rush to leave. As soon as the pace of class slows down, they roll up their mat and scurry out of the room, hoping to be first to the showers and get on with their day. People like this might get out more quickly, but they cheat themselves out of the part of the workout that engages their "brake pedal"—the rest and digest part of their nervous system that helps to make them more sound in mind and flexible in body. Two key ingredients of a cooldown are the stretches and breathing. If people don't take the time to stretch, they risk physical injury, and if they don't take time to close their mouths and breathe through their nostrils, they will likely be quick to do their feelings and use their words destructively.

The next two stages of this book are where things get wildly good! Don't forget, this is the cooldown portion. There's no striving into this part of the book, only lots of believing. True to any good cooldown, these chapters will stretch you and they will feel good. There will be parts of remaining chapters that will feel too good to be true and hard to believe. Sounds like God to me! He's giving you revelation—your body revelation. It's in this portion you will complete the transformation of your pain from something that once made you bitter to something that makes you better. It has everything to do with your thoughts, feelings, and choices as a person of faith, and your faith is fueled by your identity and privileges in Christ.

To give you a better sense of our standing as God's children, let me tell you about the primary place I go to work out. Though sometimes I move my body at home, most often I go to the gym down the street, where I must agree to their regulations to use their facility. These rules have been put in place so everyone who attends the gym can enjoy the amenities and keep the equipment in good working order. By agreeing to abide by their rules and pay my monthly dues, I become a member of the gym's community.

This gym offers me access to equipment I could never afford or fit in my home, including full-sized basketball and racquetball courts, a weight room staffed with personal trainers, a state-of-the-art group fitness studio complete with mood lighting, and highly trained and sometimes over-caffeinated group fitness instructors. I also have access to a steam room, jacuzzi, sauna, and lap pool.

My membership is confirmed by a bar code on my phone. When I place my phone in front of a little black orb at the front desk, a picture of me comes up so the woman sitting behind the desk can verify my identity. She smiles, scans my face to confirm it's me, and bang, I'm in. Whether I want to take a stretch class, lift weights, sit in the sauna, or read my Bible in the café, my grown-up playground time can begin! My identification proves I am someone who has agreed to the gym's guidelines. I belong. I am in.

According to the apostle Paul, people who put their faith in Jesus Christ belong to His Kingdom, His family, and His community. Their identity as children of God gives them access to their Father and the amenities of His Kingdom.

> The Spirit himself bears witness with our spirit that we are
> children of God, and if children, then heirs—heirs of God and
> fellow heirs with Christ, provided we suffer with him in order that
> we may also be glorified with him.
> ROMANS 8:16-17

Notice that we don't just receive a new identity as a child of God (which is pretty stinking amazing on its own). We also inherit all the resources, rights, and privileges of being royal children of a Father, the King over everything. And we aren't just heirs of God, but co-heirs with Christ, which means we can access the power of the Kingdom of God as we think, feel, and choose in our bodies—even when we suffer. This is the same power that Christ had when He was on earth.

Don't overlook the fact that Jesus, the Son of God, was neglected, misunderstood, dishonored, spit upon, abused, and crucified. He endured pain, and yet He did not sin. He refused to allow the enemy to confuse Him about His identify as the beloved Son of God. Remembering who He belonged to enabled Jesus to think, feel, and choose in line with His Father's Kingdom, even when Satan tried to sever His connection with His Father.

House Rules

Our faith in Jesus gives us belonging and access to something even better than a state-of-the-art gym complete with all the tools needed to whip our bodies into shape. We belong to God's Kingdom where we receive everything we need for godly living, overflowing with joy and giving away the love and kindness we've received.

Just as we agree to pay fees and follow certain regulations when we join our local gym, so we must abide by some house rules as members of God's Kingdom. These, too, are designed for everyone's benefit:

1. **Love God.** As children of God, we give our love and allegiance first and foremost to God Himself. Our highest affections and attention must be on God, our Father. We are to love Him as He loves us. He does so, not out of duty but delight, and this is how we are to love Him. God saw us in our orphan-like misery, eternally stuck in a vicious cycle of sin. He came to us and chose us, giving us access to all He has through His death and resurrection. There is no greater love than God's love for us. In our present body-home, the number one house rule is to love God and remain in that love. His love never quits! There's no better place to be.

2. **Love others as we love ourselves.** This one is trickier. We all go astray here. Our backstories may have prevented us from ever knowing a love like God's. We will not love others unless we love ourselves, and everything we learn about that must come from God. When we have a hard time loving ourselves or others, we

must default to house rule number one, pressing into the love of God to get from Him the love we are having a hard time giving to others.

The apostle Peter, a man of great faith and great failings, explains how God, though Christ's sacrifice, empowers us to love in this way:

Your life is a journey you must travel with a deep consciousness of God. It cost God plenty to get you out of that dead-end, empty-headed life you grew up in. He paid with Christ's sacred blood. . . . It's because of this sacrificed Messiah, whom God then raised from the dead and glorified, that you trust God, that you know you have a future in God. Now that you've cleaned up your lives by following the truth, love one another as if your lives depended on it.

1 PETER 1:18-19, 21-22, MSG

3. **Recognize that grace pays our membership fee.** Unlike an annual paid membership to the gym, our membership into God's Kingdom was neither paid by us nor will it expire. Jesus gave His life to pay our dues so we could belong to our Father's Kingdom forever! Everything we need for a healthy and whole life is in found in Him, not the world. In a sense, we all began life feeling like orphans, with an inner hunger nothing and no one could completely satisfy. That old orphan spirit will show up from time to time, trying to convince us that we aren't worthy and that God isn't trustworthy or good. Orphans are inclined to think they must do something to earn love, attention, and access to resources. But people can't earn what they already have. God's grace gives us everything we long for.

People can't earn what they already have. God's grace gives us everything we long for.

---

4. **Share good things.** As sons and daughters of God, we have access to all that is in His Kingdom so we can bring more of it to earth. God's children don't get caught up in favoritism, assuming God's goodwill is just for them. Grace is also for those who have hurt us and contributed to our pain. God wants others to be a part of His family too. As part of our divine destiny, we all can uniquely tell others about the goodness of God. We are not to keep from others what we have. God's kids share everything.

Being a child of God is better than any scannable ID, giving us access to everything we need for godly living. Our actions, words, and attitudes— especially when we face adversity—are how we make our Father in heaven seen.

> In the same way, let your light shine before others, so that they may see your good works and give glory to your Father who is in heaven.
> MATTHEW 5:16

Few things frustrate me more than heading to the gym, only to discover that my phone battery has died, cutting off access to the app that gets me into the gym. Likewise, when trouble comes our way, we can feel disconnected from our Father and His Kingdom. When that happens to you, take a moment to breathe to prevent your hypervigilant limbic brain from taking over. Remember who you are, come to yourself to come to God, and turn the other cheek. People living with a coherent mind-body connection never forget who and whose they are. They are God's sons or daughters. They belong to God for the purposes of heaven on earth, which includes metabolizing their pain so they can think, feel, and make choices as heirs of God's Kingdom.

Metabolize

Mind

1. What does having an orphan spirit mean to you?
2. How would life in your body, regarding your body, change if you lived like a child of God?

3. Which of the four "house rules" in God's Kingdom (see page 187) is hardest for you?

Mouth

Father, thank You for not leaving me as an orphan. You see the mess of my sin, and yet You still choose to be with me. Thank You for never giving up on me or leaving me. Help me understand what it means to be Your child. Help me understand how that changes everything about how I think, feel, and choose, without fear and striving, especially about my body. As Your child, I know You want me to love well using the body You have given me. Help me love You most so I can love myself and others with the same love You give me. In Jesus' name, I evict the orphan spirit and close the door to it. It can no longer find room and board in me. I am a child of God, an heir of God and a co-heir with Christ. Amen.

Move

Take ten minutes to listen to this Be Still and Be Loved meditation: https://www.revelationwellness.org/tbr/still/. Sometime today, lace up your shoes and spend twenty minutes moving while listening to this: https://www.revelationwellness.org/tbr/move/.

CHAPTER 18

YOUR NEW REALITY

THERE I WAS, THE WIFE TO ONE MAN for ten years and the mother of two young kids. I fully believed that Jesus is the way, the truth, and the life. So why—other than going to church and having Christian friends—wasn't I experiencing new life? And why did the truth of God's Word feel more like a sturdy weapon to clobber my atheist husband with than an instrument of deep personal transformation?

What's wrong with me? That became my daily groan.

After discovering the ACE study we learned about in chapter 5, I began to understand how my home environment growing up, as well as the lack of safety and attachment I'd felt to my mother and father, had negatively affected my outlook on life and the development of my brain. Hugs had been earned rather than freely given, and kind words had been a commodity to be traded. As a result, it was hard to trust others, experience God's unconditional love, and see Him at work in and around me. The executive functioning and reasoning part of my brain was weak as well.

I knew something had to change. I got to work with God, seeking to remove the obstacles that came with my pain. I started therapy, read God's Word regularly, and practiced biblical meditation to let my mind breathe and process all I was learning. I stopped using my workouts to escape and was kinder to myself. I was also more curious about what I was feeling and what my body needed from day to day.

Nonetheless, things didn't immediately get better at home. My marriage was barely holding together as the enemy seemed to keep my husband in an atheist choke hold. I relied heavily on my faith community and hoarded intercessory prayer. If prayer was offered, I took it! I can't tell you how many sweaty bosoms I wept in at church. I was shameless and desperate for change.

The greatest catapult of my healing occurred when I learned about forgiveness and its importance to God. (We will talk more about this topic in the next chapter.) But here's the thing: When you stop to think about it, releasing someone who has wronged you by forgiving them is so radical. It's not natural for people living in a natural world. But as children of God, we are born again into a new Kingdom that belongs to Him. And God's Kingdom is not a bedtime story or a fairy tale. It is supernatural, super-seding and surpassing the natural laws of this world.

As a child of God, we live (think, feel, and choose) from a new, higher reality—one in which everything proceeds from faith. Faith doesn't operate according to our timeline and rules. It is, however, the powerful perspective from which we must think, feel, and chose to live. If we don't, our bodies won't work according to God's good design. The apostle Paul explains the role of faith in our lives like this: "We are always of good courage. We know that while we are at home in the body we are away from the Lord, for we walk by faith, not by sight" (2 Corinthians 5:6-7).

Children of God, given good bodies by God, are to live according to faith, not putting ultimate confidence in what we can see. That's why I believe before considering the things we can count and measure to improve our health, like reps and calories, we must remember that we belong to God's unseen Kingdom, which operates differently from this world. Jesus made this clear when the Jewish leaders brought Him to Pilate, demanding that Jesus be executed. Uncertain of why the leaders had condemned Jesus, Pilate asked Him whether He was the King of the Jews.

Jesus answered, "My kingdom is not of this world. If my kingdom were of this world, my servants would have been fighting, that I might not be delivered over to the Jews. But my kingdom is not from the world."

JOHN 18:36

Mind-Blowing Mysteries of the Unseen World

I don't pretend to be a physicist, but other than Scripture, quantum mechanics has done more to help me understand the Kingdom Jesus was referring to than anything else. One of the most replicated and repeated studies in quantum mechanics is the double-slit experiment. I won't go into all the details, but I highly encourage you to look it up online and get ready to have your mind blown.[1] A quick and much simplified synopsis of the experiment is this: Shoot marbles (*objects* you can see) through two slits into a wall, and as you would expect, the marbles leave a dented pattern on the wall in the form of the two slits. If you push a wave of water (a *substance* you can see) through the two slits, the markings left on the wall will look like a line of multiple slits, also known as an interference wave pattern. Now, shoot photons, particles of light that can be seen with the naked eye, through the slits, and they don't leave markings as the marbles did. Instead, the particles leave an interference wave pattern. Rather than acting like unseen particles, in other words, the photons behave like waves.

This phenomenon baffled physicists, who had expected these subatomic particles to act like particles. In an effort to discover what was happening, they created a device to "watch" as the photons passed through the slits. What they saw left them dumbfounded. Every time the device observed what was happening, the photons acted like particles rather than waves. But whenever the measuring device wasn't watching, the particle behaved like waves again. It's so weird! It's almost as if, when the unseen world knew it was being watched, the photons acted as one would expect.[2]

Scientists have theories about why observation affects the outcome of the experiment. Is it possible that energy has a consciousness and "knows" when it's being observed? Some quantum physicists theorize that some sort of "consciousness" exists and participates with what is unseen; however, since God doesn't fit into the world of observational science, most are unlikely to attribute this consciousness to Him.

I agree with Max Planck, who is considered one of the fathers of quantum physics:

> As a man who has devoted his whole life to the most clearheaded science, to the study of matter, I can tell you as a result of my research about the atoms this much: There is no matter as such! All matter originates and exists only by virtue of a force which brings the particles of an atom to vibration and holds this most minute solar system of the atom together. . . . We must assume behind this force the existence of a conscious and intelligent Mind. This Mind is the matrix of all matter.[3]

Friends, as believers we know this "conscious and intelligent Mind" is Yahweh—the one true God. The maker of your body. The maker of heaven and earth and all creation. The Alpha. The Omega. The beginning and the end. He was there at the start when He made all things, and He will be there at the end when all earthly matters return to Him. He is the force behind the unseen that holds all seen things together. He holds your seen body *and* unseen soul together.

> For by him all things were created, in heaven and on earth,
> visible and invisible, whether thrones or dominions or rulers or
> authorities—all things were created through him and for him.
> And he is before all things, and in him all things hold together.
> COLOSSIANS 1:17

People are the crowns of God's physically seen creation, the only beings made in His image. Our bodies, physical matter consisting of muscles, bones, blood, water, and trillions of cells, are held together by the existence of an unseen God. He desires to make heaven seen on earth through us. In faith, we give Him all of our selves and, through faith, we think, feel, and choose from the powerful reality of God's Kingdom! This is not just an idea; it is a reality that wants to break into our natural world. Dallas

Willard defines it as "the range of [God's] effective will, where what he wants done is done."[4] Our bodies are the perfect vehicle for the unseen Kingdom of God's will to be done and the perfect place for this unseen Kingdom to reside.

There are several key concepts of quantum physics that we can apply to life in our physical bodies:

- Observation affects outcome.
- The unseen world is a participatory universe.
- Anything is possible in the unseen world.

1. **Observation affects outcome.** My interpretation of the double-slit experiment is that when the unseen world knows it's being monitored, it refuses to do impossible things like changing into another form (e.g., a particle won't move as a wave does). On the other hand, when no longer observed, subatomic particles like photons and electrons often act like waves.[5]

   Likewise, in the Bible we read about God's Spirit transforming people in supernatural ways. Joseph, Moses, Esther, Daniel, Mary, and Peter are just a few examples of those who went from being ordinary to extraordinary people, saying and doing incredibly courageous things. I suggest that God wants to do a new work in you as well—immeasurably more than you can ask, imagine, or *see* kind of work. However, consistently limiting yourself to what you can see, measure, or experience affects your ability to access God's reality, the power of His unseen Kingdom, which you now belong to and represent as a child of God. Faith, which "is being sure of what we hope for and certain of what we do not see" (Hebrews 11:1), enables us to become active participants in God's Kingdom.

   When we base our expectation only on what we can physically observe, see, hear, feel, taste, touch, or measure in inches, pounds, or calories, we interfere with the unseen world from which faith operates. The door to the Kingdom of God closes. In other words, when we think, talk, or act without faith, we interfere with the Kingdom's operation, power, and transforming possibilities. We are thinking, feeling, and choosing in accordance with the prince of this world, Satan, who wants to keep us out of the presence of God so we can't access the peace and power found in God's unseen Kingdom. On the other hand, if we choose to observe all things, including negative circumstances, from the unseen perspective of faith, the door to God's boundless and surprising Kingdom opens to us as His children.

When we base our expectation only on what we can physically observe, see, hear, feel, taste, touch, or measure in inches, pounds, or calories, we interfere with the unseen world from which faith operates.

Choosing to live by faith doesn't mean we can ignore the facts of poor health. Instead, we don't give those facts the final say. In faith, we partner with God until we see the facts change. When someone promotes a diet or other product that they promise will melt away the pounds so we can be model thin (and thus worthy of others' love and admiration), we shut our eyes and ears. We turn away from what the world tells us our bodies should look like and keep taking steps forward with God. Yes, we face our fears and pain, which may mean changing the way we eat and move, but we do so in order to think, feel, and choose like Him. Every step we take in faith, according to His Word, helps heal our tired bodies, mend our broken hearts, rewire our brains, and renew our minds so we can observe the Kingdom of God affecting the reality of earth.

2. **The unseen world is a participatory universe.** Since I think the unseen world seems to know when someone is "watching" it, I believe it also appears open for partnership. The unseen world of

faith, where anything is possible, is looking for a friend who wants to play. But the unseen world will play with us only if we abide by one rule: Don't ruin the fun by keeping score. Our earthbound formulas of $1 + 2 = 3$, or $A + B = C$, don't work when playing in the sandbox of faith. As we just learned, measuring reality by our standards shuts down the operation of faith, which is required if we are to live from and access God's Kingdom here on earth. When Jesus invites us to take His yoke upon us and learn from Him (Matthew 11:29), He's looking for friends to plow and play in the field of faith with Him. Just don't ruin the fun and slow down the game by picking up a heavy yoke of earthbound rules like keeping score and measuring everything.

3. **Anything is possible in the unseen world as long as we have faith.** When Jesus' disciples couldn't cast out a demon from a boy, Jesus admonished them for their lack of faith: "Truly, I say to you, if you have faith like a grain of mustard seed, you will say to this mountain, 'Move from here to there,' and it will move, and nothing will be impossible for you" (Matthew 17:20). Nothing will be impossible for us, Jesus? Really? Quantum physics shows that this is absolutely true!

   I like to think that Jesus chose to partner with the reality of quantum physics when He went through walls, walked on water, healed the sick, and raised the dead. He could do these supernatural things because He knew who He was and what He was on earth to do. He was the Son of God, the substance of pure faith that moves mountains, sent to show us His Father's Kingdom.

   In the unseen world of pure faith, anything is possible and nothing is predictable. That means we shouldn't limit the possibilities of faith by predicting or measuring outcomes. This form of judgment is something people who are mindful of God's Kingdom don't do. Only God in His purity and holiness is worthy of having the final say over everyone and everything. People who live from the reality of God's unseen Kingdom believe and pray boldly for God-pleasing outcomes. We never predict or pray for an outcome according to worldly standards, and we realize that challenges are a part of life. When we pray for outcomes that will please God's heart, we keep the door of faith open to His Kingdom, where unlimited opportunities and possibilities exist.

In the unseen world of pure faith,
anything is possible and nothing is predictable.

"In the beginning, God" (Genesis 1:1). He is the goodness and consciousness that's always been. It's from God that we live, move, and have our being. And in His Kingdom, who we are is more unseen (energy) than seen (matter).

So let's keep our ears open to God's Word and our eyes closed to the standards of the world, including man-made ideals like the optimal body shape or size and what our fitness ability should be. If we are going to transform our aches and pains into purposes that give God glory and bring us joy, we must never forget who we are and what we have. We are God's chosen children with access to His eternal Kingdom where no problems exist, only endless possibilities. Our pain can be transformed into purpose as long as we walk by faith and not by sight. Let's leave behind our earthbound orphan spirit that judges, weighs, and measures everything. If we can't see it today, that doesn't mean we won't someday.

Metabolize

Mind

1. How does the reality of an unseen world that doesn't operate like the seen world change the way you view your body and health?
2. If you were to partner with faith (the unseen world) when you feel pain, what would that look like?
3. Do a Google search for "Bible verses about faith." After reading several passages, answer this question: What does God want you to know about faith?

Mouth

God, I was blind, but now I see. Your Kingdom is a reality that proceeds from faith. Anything is possible with You. I want to constantly be sure of what I hope for and certain of what I do not see. If what I see is not in line with You or Your Kingdom from which righteousness, peace, and joy flow (Romans 14:17), renew my mind and set me free. Come, Holy Spirit. The pain I've lived through has disrupted the peaceful connection between my brain and heart and kept me from living in the reality of Your unseen Kingdom. Take these negative feelings and remind me that nothing is impossible for You. Help me to be content in all things, knowing that there is no lack in your Kingdom. Rather than seeing problems, teach me to recognize the unlimited possibilities so Your Kingdom can continue to move through me. Help me observe what's going on around and in me without judging what I feel, hear, or see. Amen.

Move

Build a Boat

Like Noah, build a B.O.A.T. The next time you begin to feel emotional pain, try this faith exercise so you can continue living from your new reality.

B (breathe): Once you notice you're not feeling, thinking, or choosing well, begin to purposely breathe. Inhale for the count of five, and exhale for the count of five. Aim to take nine breaths in ninety seconds. Fire up your parasympathetic nervous system (brake pedal) as the chemicals designed to keep you safe (e.g., cortisol, adrenaline) are released in your brain and then run their course through your body.

O (observe): As you breathe, take a moment to step back from the circumstance and simply notice what's going on. Observe the moment without judgment by tapping into your ability to be mindful. This will help activate the higher reasoning of your MPFC.

A (acknowledge): Don't be rude to your feelings. Recognize those feelings. Name them under your breath if you need to. *I am so mad* or *I am* *disappointed* are honest feelings that need to be felt. Just keep in mind that while feelings are real, they aren't truth. But feelings have the ability to lead you to the God who is Truth, the One who can help you in your time of need.

T (transform): By faith, transform what you are feeling to be congruent with God's Word and what He wants to do in your life. For example, if you're feeling disappointed because you didn't get the job promotion you were praying for, by faith call on God. Remember that you are praying "to him who is able to do immeasurably more than all we ask or imagine, according to his power that is at work within us" (Ephesians 3:20, NIV). Have faith that God is bringing you something better, then go about your day living that way!

Take ten minutes to listen to this Be Still and Be Loved meditation, which goes along with what you've just read: https://www.revelation wellness.org/tbr/still/. Then sometime today, lace up your shoes and move for twenty minutes while listening to this audio recording: https://www .revelationwellness.org/tbr/move/.

CHAPTER 19

FORGIVENESS AND THE PARTY POOPERS

GIVE IT TO ME, ALISA. It's much too heavy for you to carry.

I heard the Holy Spirit whisper these words over and over again.

I didn't want to let it go. After ten years of living through the pain and what felt like the agony of being married to a man who didn't love God and seemed only to tolerate me, I was stuck. I was stuck in unforgiveness. I was stuck but felt safe behind the walls I had built.

We live in a world that's fractured due to sin, which means things won't always go the way we know they should. Children should be able to trust that their parents will love them, care for them, and lead them well. Friends should be confident that they won't stab one another in the back. And when people commit themselves to another for life with an "I do," they should mean what they say and do it, even when they don't feel like it. But our hearts are deceitful because of sin. We don't always do what we should. And when things don't go the way we think they should, we feel loss—namely a loss of control over our lives. When we feel as if we have lost control, we are likely to retreat into safety and survival mode. Unforgiveness becomes a state of being. It's like a bomb shelter we run to when hurt, but once there, we are locked in. What felt like a safe space becomes a prison. We may feel emotionally safe, but we are physically stuck.

Sarah grew up in a home with an alcoholic mother who struggled with mental health issues. Her dad had left when Sarah was young. As a result, Sarah carried the burden of caring for her mom as far back as she can remember. Her childhood didn't look like that of other kids on the block. Between going to school and looking for ways to earn money to help support them, Sarah doesn't remember much about being a kid. "I was always working," she told me. Sarah did everything she could to suppress her resentment and the silent rage that burned within. By the time she was thirty, Sarah's health was beginning to fail. It started with skin and digestive issues and eventually led to a thyroid condition. Because her doctor and the specialists he sent her to couldn't find a reason for her pain, she was diagnosed with an autoimmune disease. (That meant she was expected to live with pain for which there was no cure, only a medication that might keep it under control.)

After being told she would battle this condition for the rest of her life, Sarah was determined to work on her health by eating clean and joining a gym, where she went several times a week. She also started going to therapy. One day she sensed the Holy Spirit telling her, *Sarah, you can change your food all you want, but your healing and wholeness will come through forgiveness.* Sarah dropped to her knees on her kitchen floor. Right there and then she experienced a radical encounter of forgiveness. She released both her mother and her father for what they had done and hadn't done. Sarah later told me, "It didn't change them in that moment, but it did change me."

A year after that holy moment on her kitchen floor, her lab work showed no sign of her disease. The physical pain she'd felt ceased. One year after that, her mom passed away from cancer. "Before she left this earth," Sarah said, "I was able to say to her with my whole heart, it is well with my soul." Forgiveness didn't just bring health to Sarah's soul but to her whole body too.

Sarah's experience lines up with the science. According to John Hopkins Medicine, "the act of forgiveness can reap huge rewards for your health, lowering the risk of heart attack; improving cholesterol levels and sleep; and reducing pain, blood pressure, and levels of anxiety, depression and stress. And research points to an increase in the forgiveness-health connection as you age."[1] Notice that reducing pain is one of the rewards of forgiveness.

Let's think about how feelings associated with unforgiveness affect our bodies. The body experiences the emotions of anger or resentment as stress, which results in a tightening and tensing of the body. The emotional energy behind anger tells our body to close down rather than open up. For example, a man who is angry and wants to hit someone doesn't open his hands to clap and cheer. No, he closes his hands and makes a fist. A woman who is angry doesn't open her eyes and mouth in joy and surprise but purses her lips tightly with a furrowed brow and squinting eyes.

When we hold on to this anger and resentment, we experience chronic stress. And as we now know, ongoing stress disrupts the organization and operation of our brain, making it difficult to reason and to think, feel, and choose what's best. Furthermore, our bodies can't fully heal. As dearly loved children of God, we should want the cells of our body to open up to God's healing presence rather than close down in anger, resentment, or hate. If we really want our bodies and souls to be well, accessing the power for healing and transforming pain is contingent upon our ability to forgive.

Don't Miss the Party

The cost of unforgiveness goes even deeper. Jesus told His followers, "If you forgive others their trespasses, your heavenly Father will also forgive you, but if you do not forgive others their trespasses, neither will your Father forgive your trespasses" (Matthew 6:14-15).

Did you catch that? If you refuse to forgive, Jesus said, "Neither will I."

Because they've been forgiven, Christians have been given a key to their Father's Kingdom. According to Matthew 6:14-15, however, it's possible to believe in Jesus yet have keys that won't work. When we struggle to forgive someone—even though we know we've been called to do so and want to obey God—we won't be able to access the power and resources of God's Kingdom. We're stuck in a standoff with God. Stuck but safe.

The Greek word *aphiēmi*, translated "forgive" here, can mean "to send away," "to let go," "to give up," or "to leave behind."[2] To forgive, in other words, means to let go. I don't know about you, but my initial instinct is *not* to let someone go who's wronged me. My natural reaction is to keep an account of the wrongs done, including details that support my version of what happened, my role as the victim and theirs as the problem that needs to be fixed. I then begin crafting a list of things this person must do before I forgive them (if I ever will).

The problem: If we don't let go of the wrongs we've done or the wrongs done to us, God won't free us. God is serious about His people living coherent and integrated lives in which they give away forgiveness as freely as they've been given it. If we don't forgive, it will be impossible for us to live from the reality of our Father's Kingdom where we have everything we need. Remember the elder brother who was unforgiving toward his rebellious younger brother, the Prodigal Son? His father urged him to let go of his resentment by remembering all the gifts he'd been given: "And he said to him, 'Son, you are always with me, and all that is mine is yours'" (Luke 15:31). When we hold on to unforgiveness as he did, we will find it difficult to move freely and joyfully through life representing God's marvelous Kingdom.

Jesus told the parable of the Prodigal Son in an attempt to help the religious leaders better understand God's extravagant grace, which includes His desire that we forgive others as well. Earlier we looked at Matthew 6:14-15, where Jesus tells us He will not forgive us if we refuse to forgive others. This passage is part of the Sermon on the Mount, Jesus' explanation of what the Kingdom of God is like and how the people of God are to live.

His message in both Matthew 6 and Luke 15 disrupted everything the religious people—with their overactive, amygdala-driven brains— knew about God. The Kingdom Jesus introduced is counterintuitive and countercultural to the world's ways. In God's Kingdom, the way up is down. You're blessed when you have nothing. The meek, not the strong, are given the world.

Humility was not valued in my home growing up, and my parents never told me "I'm sorry." While it would have meant so much to hear my mom or dad recognize when they'd hurt me, I now realize that even saying "I am sorry" is not really the same as asking for forgiveness. It's an important acknowledgment, but on its own it doesn't go far enough. It's a statement based on me with *I* as the subject. On the other hand, asking someone,

"Will you forgive me?" is a question that invites another's participation. Inviting someone to release you from your wrongdoing requires humility because asking for forgiveness is riskier than making a personal statement of regret. Asking for forgiveness means seeking a radical act of mercy and grace from someone. It's a gift from the Kingdom of God for the miserable and afflicted.

Saying "I am sorry" is not really the same as asking for forgiveness. On the other hand, asking someone, "Will you forgive me?" invites another's participation.

Maybe more importantly, giving and receiving mercy and grace through forgiveness keeps the gospel alive and well in our hearts and on planet earth. Giving and receiving forgiveness shows the world we are genuine followers of Jesus, not just believers in Jesus. We have a faith that's backed by action, rooted in humility. Our faith has feet! When we exercise forgiveness, we do what people who live according to their flesh find impossible to do. We also make the unseen power of God's Kingdom seen and attractive to those who are perishing. And bonus! We bring healing to our bodies and bones too!

Three years ago as I'm writing this, my mother passed away from ovarian cancer. And one year ago, my father passed away from complications related to prostate cancer. When cleaning out my parents' house, I found many notes my mother wrote about her hurts, including this one about my dad:

> Eddie believes that whatever wrong he did in our family that he is not to blame for our behavior. I disagree. He should have made amends to all of us, by actions.

The note she left behind is evidence of the pain my mom lived with. That pain kept her brain and body stuck, living in the valley of fight, flight, or freeze, looking for someone to blame and creating a checklist of all my dad needed to do before he could enter back into her graces.

Thank God He is not like us. He is rich in mercy and grace. His desire to set us free from the wear and tear sin makes on our bodies, brains, hearts, and souls never runs out!

I did not want my marriage to end up like my parents'. As I experienced God's mercy and grace toward me in a deeper way, God continued to work on and heal me. I started to respond to my overactive amygdala with kindness and curiosity about what I was feeling and thinking. With the help of the Holy Spirit, I became a responder rather than a reactor to pain. I became more compassionate and empathetic toward myself and then toward others. Once I was kinder to myself and relied more upon God to meet my needs, my heart softened toward Simon. At that point, Simon's heart softened toward God. Our marriage began to mend, and forgiveness flowed more naturally between us. The love of Jesus was at work in our home and by God's grace, after ten years of prodigal living, Simon came back to himself. He realized how foolish it was to fight against my heart, which wanted only good for him and for others, as was evident in Revelation Wellness, the ministry God began through me. Simon laid down his weapons and in humility came home to the Lord. After fifteen turbulent years, our marriage was moving into new territory—a place of unity and peace. The love of God really does give us the ability to endure all things—along with the ability to respond with kindness and patience as we wait.

In challenging moments when circumstances don't look bright, people with the mind of Christ default to trusting God; they are more aware of the unseen than the seen. Forgiveness is their default mode so they "assume the best" of others, which activates the empathy area of their brain. This enables them to see others as fellow image bearers of God who have also experienced pain. Research shows that optimistic thinking improves our mental and physical health.[3] It's as if God really did design us to be at our best when we're loving and forgiving.

A person who lives in freedom processes stress differently, knowing that in God's Kingdom there is no lack and anything is possible. As citizens of the abundant Kingdom, God's people are quick to extend mercy, grace, and forgiveness when they are wronged. As soon as they recognize they have wronged another, they are quick to acknowledge it and seek forgiveness. They recognize that feelings aren't facts and can obstruct the flow of freedom. This, my brother and sister, is why we train physically *and* spiritually! Physical training—whether stretching, lifting heavy weights, or moving continuously through space—makes time for the body to talk to the mind. In physicality we manifest what we believe spiritually—that we are comfortable being uncomfortable and believe that accepting challenges like forgiving even when we don't feel like it produces change. Physical and spiritual training with God at the center makes us congruent beings—people who have faith in God (spiritual), do our faith (physical), and refuse to be ruled by our feelings (emotional).

In our modern world of convenience, we can outsource hard work with one click. Need groceries? Instacart to the rescue. Need school supplies? Amazon's got your back. But one thing we can't outsource is our bodies. We must do the work. When stress comes, we have to purposefully settle our bodies down to breathe through the tension. Or we might release the strain by going for a walk or run. People of God get physical to stay integrated in their bodies and minds, and they go to God to find freedom from carrying or causing unnecessary pain. They recognize that forgiveness will lead to freedom—for themselves, just as much as for those who have wronged them.

The Party Poopers

Not everyone who loves God and wants to love others well will be free and forgiving. When the rebellious Prodigal Son returned home, his father insisted on throwing an extravagant celebration to welcome him back. In Luke 15, we read about one person who was not eager to party. After returning from another day of working his father's fields, the older son heard the preparations being made. This was the brother who had kept all the rules and lived a tidy life. Now he was very disgruntled and displeased with his younger brother: "He was angry and refused to go in" (Luke 15:28). The elder brother was a party pooper. Nothing about his father's kindness and forgiveness made sense to him. Stress and bitterness flooded his heart, blocking love and empathy.

How much relief he might have felt had he chosen to spend more time with his father, enjoying his company rather than distracting himself from his anger and trying to prove his worthiness to his father through his toil in the field. Unwilling to process his anger and hurt, he apparently believed that hard work was the way to deal with his agitation.

While his reaction may seem understandable on the surface, the older brother's unforgiving spirit was obstructing the full expression of grace meant to flow from his father's goodness. As children of God, we are meant to let His good news move and flow freely, especially in the face of adversity when it is most needed. We don't want to obstruct others' view of God because we are stuck in unforgiveness. God's power is displayed most vividly in our moments of weakness, allowing those who are hurting to see something in us that they need. As we learned in the last chapter, living this way is possible when we walk by faith and not by sight. As the observers and participants of God's unseen Kingdom, we know we are to avoid judging outcomes and other people because that obstructs God's flow of mercy and grace and the unlimited potential and possibilities of His Kingdom.

Like moving your body and eating well, learning to forgive is a daily practice. Truthfully, forgiveness is not something that comes from us anyway. As citizens of God's Kingdom, we don't belong to the world but to God's family. Rather than relying on the world's broken justice system, we are to trust God, our Father, the Maker of heaven and earth, to right all wrongs according to His higher ways, on His time, and in His economy. We are absolutely called to seek justice (Micah 6:8), but we can't fall into the trap of judgment. As God's children, we are to bring healing to broken things with the love of God, whose mercy triumphs over judgment. God wants to bring more of His goodness to earth through us. Living judgmentally with unforgiveness for ourselves or another who caused us pain is an obstacle to God's loving-kindness and healing ways.

We are absolutely called to seek justice (Micah 6:8),
but we can't fall into the trap of judgment.

As you continue to live free in body and soul, metabolizing your pain into purpose, be aware of the party poopers. Your promotion to seeing as God sees will lead to better thinking, feeling, and choosing regarding your health. But it will feel like a demotion to those who see as the world does. They live as my mother did: hard on themselves and others. Such people need your love and empathy.

I confess that, for most of my life, I was critical of my mom. I blamed her for being so hard on me and for not being strong enough to leave my father and stand on her own two feet. I judged her for not loving and trusting in the God she said she believed in. It wasn't until the last few months of her life when I held her hand and watched her body wither away that all that nonsense faded away. Forgiveness poured out like a river overflowing with goodbye tears. She left my life forgiven and free, and I had more space in my soul to breathe. Now she's a legend in my book. Love and forgiveness have the power to rewrite our stories of pain. Don't wait another day for your better story. Forgive.

Initially you may find it very hard to forgive some people because they don't feel safe. Keep in mind that forgiveness doesn't necessarily lead to reconciliation. Forgiveness is for letting the person go and for us to stop "playing God" by judging. Then you get out of God's way and see what happens.

You are loved by God and forgiven. You are free! So stay free. Exercise gracious assumptions while keeping healthy boundaries. Pray for those you need to forgive. Bless them. Love sacrificially. You don't have to let party poopers into your personal freedom party unless they, too, are willing to listen, learn, and forgive. They are still your neighbors, people to love and forgive, even if they refuse to love and forgive you. Show them the beauty of God's unseen Kingdom.

If you want to be someone who can process pain into good purpose and live in good health as far as it depends on you, you must learn to let go freely and forgive. As you live in the freedom that forgiveness provides, you will delightfully discover how freely and lightly you can move!

Metabolize

Mind

1. Who or what comes to mind when you hear the word *forgive*?
2. How might unforgiveness be playing a role in your physical health?

Mouth

God, thank You for forgiving me. I want to live, love, and freely forgive like Jesus. Please help me, Holy Spirit, to be a person who actively forgives as soon as I feel hurt. I know I am prone to run to the bomb shelter of unforgiveness instead, but I want to live lightly and freely. I want to graciously assume the best of everyone rather than thinking suspiciously. Thank You, God, that this is a work You want and will do in me. I believe! Amen.

Move

Train for forgiveness! The next time you wrong another, don't just say "I'm sorry." Therapists and marriage counselors Dr. Don and Renee Worcester played a big role in helping me learn how to ask for forgiveness. It looks like this:

1. **Humble yourself.** When feeling the weight of wrongdoing, humble yourself. Ask God for His forgiveness and then freely receive it. But don't stop there. Give the enemy of freedom a black eye by going to the other person and asking for forgiveness. In other words, subdue and have dominion over a spirit of unforgiveness. Clean up your mess and "take out the trash." Start the conversation with "I would like to ask your forgiveness for something I've done. Is this a good time?" Usually, this statement will disarm anyone who has something against us. That's the power of humility. The person you are asking forgiveness from has the right to say no. Just know that it's in the process of going to and asking God and another for forgiveness that you're free. If they don't want to forgive you, they are the ones who are stuck—not you. Continue to pray for them to be set free and for the enemy who is holding them captive to go back to hell. You were set free when you humbled yourself before God and that person by asking for forgiveness. Now stay free. Don't play the enemy's game and take on a spirit of condemnation or shame. Stay sober minded; keep watch and pray.

2. **Confess.** If the person is receptive to hearing your apology, you can say, "I would like to ask your forgiveness for _____." Don't

say any more than that. No adding on "When you did _____, I did _____." Don't justify what you did and why you did it. If they go off on a tangent, just listen patiently. Carry your cross and absorb the suffering as Jesus did for us. Breathe deeply and remember: This is why you train!

3. **Empathize.** Now here comes the real *Karate Kid* move. Ask them, "How did it make you feel when I _____?" Then listen to understand rather than to be understood. This is where you learn the love and empathy of Christ. Let the tears come. They come from godly sorrow that leads to repentance (2 Corinthians 7:10). You're being healed and refreshed.

4. **Request feedback.** Ask them, "How could I have done that better?" Really listen with the heart of wanting to learn to do better. This step in asking forgiveness is especially powerful and healing for people who have never felt heard in their pain.

5. **Ask for freedom through forgiveness.** Once you've listened as they process how your actions affected them, ask, "Will you forgive me?" Usually they will say yes. But even if they don't, remember . . . you are forgiven and free! *And* you modeled the gospel to another person in need. You can walk away from that conversation knowing you have pleased your Father's heart.

If this all seems big and scary, I encourage you to start practicing forgiveness with a child. Children live so close to the Kingdom that they are generally quick to forgive, enabling you both to get back to playing and enjoying life.

Next take ten minutes to listen to this Be Still and Be Loved meditation: https://www.revelationwellness.org/tbr/still/. Sometime today, lace up your shoes and move for twenty minutes while listening to this audio recording: https://www.revelationwellness.org/tbr/move/.

CHAPTER 20

TELLING YOURSELF
THE TRUTH

"I THINK I WOULD LIKE TO LEARN what it takes to become a police officer."

Steve's wife, Cindy, looks confused, trying to process what he just told her. "A what?"

"Yeah. I think it would be really cool! What do you think?"

Cindy's husband, a highly dependable, white-collar accountant, was asking her if he could become a volunteer police officer on the weekends. Steve wanted to risk his life on the rough streets of the city they called home.

Underneath the initial current of anxiety she felt, Cindy knew that the Holy Spirit was calling Steve back to his original design—to be the person God created him to be, not who the world or his parents told him he should be. Steve's father had encouraged him to become a certified public accountant (CPA) because accounting ran in the family. It was a natural and reasonable fit. Although Steve is the most intelligent man Cindy knows and is crazy good at everything he puts his mind to, his heart comes alive when he can serve the weak and protect the innocent.

In the summer of 2013, Steve was sworn in as a full-fledged police officer. He would serve as a reserve officer by night while remaining a CPA by day.

Cindy had married Batman. Who knew?

As a police officer, it's Steve's job to maintain order and peace on the streets. Sometimes he must arrest people doing bad things. He commands perpetrators to stop running, drop to their knees, and raise their hands to show they have no weapons. He can then safely approach the individual and put the perpetrator in handcuffs behind their back. As soon as they're constrained, it's nearly impossible for the offender to do anything.

Steve told Cindy, "It's funny. Once a suspect is under arrest and in handcuffs, they get really bold. They get mouthy and say things they wouldn't say to a police officer before being arrested. Stripped of all weapons, all they have left is their mouth."

This is just like Satan's strategy now that he has been disarmed by Jesus at the Cross. He is utterly and completely defenseless against God and His Kingdom. Because of Jesus' victory, we can worship God with all of who we are, and our authority to subdue and have dominion over the world has been restored. Let's put it in good news/bad new terminology:

Good news: Satan is disarmed; he's lost his ability to keep people
  away from the love of God.
Bad news: This defeat has made our enemy mouthier.

That's all Satan has left to use against God's children. And boy, oh boy, is he a mouthy and disrespectful one. He never shuts up.

You're fat.
You're ugly.
You're old, and nobody cares about you.
Nobody wants you—just look at yourself. You're disgusting and
  undesirable.
You have no self-control, you lazy slob.
You deserved that.
You are a terrible person.

You should have known better.
That's your problem to fix.
You should be ashamed of yourself.
No wonder your parents left you.
Since they hurt you, you should hurt them and get what you deserve.
It will never get better for you.
You're alone, and nobody cares about you anyway.

Of course Satan seeks to discourage us, tear us down, and feed us lies. It's the only tactic he has left. The apostle Paul explains the cosmic battle that disarmed our enemy:

You, who were dead in your trespasses and the uncircumcision of your flesh, God made alive together with him, having forgiven us all our trespasses, by canceling the record of debt that stood against us with its legal demands. This he set aside, nailing it to the cross. He *disarmed* the rulers and authorities and put them to open shame, by triumphing over them in him.

COLOSSIANS 2:13-15 (EMPHASIS MINE)

Of course Satan seeks to discourage us, tear us down,
and feed us lies. It's the only tactic he has left.

The Cross disarmed Satan. Meaning: He has no arms! Would you agree that our arms make it easier to get things done? The Cross neutralized Satan but it didn't shut him up. He still has use of his tongue. With it he twists what God says, hoping someone will believe and act on his lies.

Because this book is centered on our bodies, it's intriguing to think that, because of Jesus, Satan and his coworkers have no arms. One day he and his demons will be thrown into hell forever. Until then, they are like a detained person in handcuffs: For now they roam the earth looking for hurting people, those with a hostile spirit toward God, hoping to deceive them. Some people are easy targets because they have never been shown or given mercy, grace, and forgiveness. With their hurting hearts and minds, they easily believe Satan's lies. And with their bodies and their hands, they can do Satan's dirty work for him.

Though people who have no relationship with God are easy targets, I suspect that Satan takes special delight when he sees Christ followers fall for one of his obnoxious lies. When we believe the evil one's mouthy lies, we, too, become his hands—his tool to hurt more people. To live as people who transform pain into purpose and trouble into triumph, who steward our bodies to bring more heaven to earth, we must stop allowing ourselves to be taken in by the enemy. How do we stop his violent abuse of our minds?

> We destroy arguments and every lofty opinion raised against the knowledge of God, and take every thought captive to obey Christ.
>
> 2 CORINTHIANS 10:5

When we do this, we keep the enemy disarmed. We keep him in on his knees and handcuffed at the foot of the Cross, submitting to Jesus. When we take captive every thought the devil tries to plant in us, we kick him back to his rightful place, powerless in God's Kingdom. We are then free to take out the trash of lies and suspicions about our good bodies, our Good Father, and His plans for us in His Kingdom.

What are we to do with those lies that we find especially difficult to take captive? Recurrent, destructive thoughts don't just need to be taken captive; they need their day in court.

Putting Our Thoughts on Trial

When Steve arrests someone, he detains that person by putting them in handcuffs. He then slides them into the back of his cop car and heads to the local jail, where the suspect is booked. The booking records the details of the suspected offense, but this doesn't mean the suspect is guilty of a crime. If the offense that the suspect allegedly committed is not egregious, the person can post bail after a short time behind bars. Bail is meant to assure that the suspect will return for their day in court where a judge or jury will determine whether they are guilty of whatever they're being accused of.

Let's apply the above scenario to see why we struggle as Christ followers to cultivate a healthy thought life.

1. **Surface survival living.** We are so busy building our kingdom here on earth that we fail to take our thoughts captive to make them obedient to Christ. Rather than being transformed by the words of God and allowing Him to make purpose of our pain, we survive by hiding behind the Word of God while keeping busy doing "good." We go to church. We read our Bibles. On the surface we keep our lives tidy and clean.

   But all our busyness keeps us from the business of tending to the condition of our souls. We need margin and space in our days to be with God and spend less time doing things for God. (And again . . . some of us like to say that studying the Bible is the same as being with God. But if our studying isn't producing the fruit of kind words and actions, we may be too much like the elder brother who was so busy working that he didn't appreciate his father's grace.) You need more time to be still (or even go for a walk and talk) with God and be loved.

   All our busyness keeps us from the business
   of tending to the condition of our souls.

   ---

2. **Imposter syndrome.** Because negative thoughts don't feel good, we quickly try to repress or cover up bad thoughts with positive words or affirmations rather than getting curious and then vigilant about challenging them. When we live in this state of ignorant bliss, we never deal with the genesis of our destructive thoughts and feelings. Surface living disconnects us from the deepest fears that drive our desires, thoughts, and feelings. With a happy face we present

ourselves to the world as "good Christians" but have a hard time loving and liking ourselves. A 2009 study showed that people who say positive things like "I am worthy of love" but don't have the positive self-esteem and mindset to back up those statements feel worse than if they hadn't spoken them at all.[1]

Saying something they don't believe can make a person feel like a fraud. And imposter syndrome can be taken to a whole other level for Christians. We declare Scripture over our lives, put verses on our walls, drink out of coffee cups inscribed with Scripture, but often fail to live according to the words we declare. And not being able to do what we believe can leave us feeling more ashamed and hopeless than people who don't believe in God. We hate falling short—not to mention the God we say we love. Letting both ourselves and God down leads to a double whammy of shame.

3. **Overcrowding.** We can't hold a wrong thought captive indefinitely. After we hold it in captivity for a few seconds, we let it go and move on to the next thought. There are only so many thoughts we can keep captive at one time. If painful thoughts keep returning, over and over, those thoughts need a day in court. Otherwise, our minds will overflow, and we will let a lot of wrong thoughts go free. These trespassing thoughts can wreak havoc on our bodies and brains. They are like fugitives with no intention of returning for their court date.

When the enemy, our accuser, continually trespasses on our minds, planting the same destructive thoughts, he needs his day in court. Jail is a temporary place where people who've been taken captive go. Court is where these captive people go so the truth can be made known and proper sentencing is handed down. I think as Christians we know how to take our thoughts captive when what we really need is a sentencing of our thoughts—a final verdict from God about the thoughts we are having.

When do you know court session is needed? When you notice that you are trying to keep disturbing thoughts on a surface level, feel like a fraud, or are taking the same thought captive repeatedly, you may need to take this step. Pay attention to your body. It is speaking, trying to keep you safe.

Notice when your stomach turns, brow furrows, hands clench, shoulders lift, or you feel short of breath. Your body is trying to tell you that something is not right. Something is not true or worthy of your attention.

First, breathe deeply. Stay in the moment, aware of your agency as a child of God. Second, take that thought captive. Disarm Satan of his weapon by calling out "Lie!" Next, take him and his stinking thinking immediately to court. (If you aren't in a place or in the headspace to take a thought to court—such as during an important work meeting—go ahead and put that thought in jail as a temporary holding place. But if you want to strengthen the coherence between your body and brain, you must make time to take that destructive recurring thought to court.)

Our thoughts are not made obedient to Christ because we took them captive and put them in jail. Our thoughts are made obedient to Christ in God's courtroom. Luckily for us, we are God's kids, so we don't have to wait long for a court date. We get immediate justice because we know the Judge. He's our Father! He's happy to show up to court anytime, day or night, to deal with the offenders who hurt His kids.

Let's practice putting a thought on trial—specifically a common lie of our enemy: "You're fat and ugly, and nobody cares about you."

This is how I picture it going down. Your attorney for this hearing is the Holy Spirit. He's your Advocate. But before going into court, He needs a private moment with you without your offender present.

Holy Spirit: "First question: When the accuser said these words, what specifically was your desire?"

Remember, your misplaced desires open you up to partnering with lies. We are designed to desire God, but we often go after other things. The lies behind our desires produce stress, and ongoing stress damages our bodies and brains. We must come clean about how those wants that don't come from God lead us to entertain lies.

You: "I was nervous about going to my work party. I just wanted to look and feel good in my clothes and was surprised when my pants didn't fit."

Second question: "What makes acquiring your desire so difficult?"
Reply: "No matter what I do, I never seem to feel good in my body.
And my work friends always look so much better than me."

Third question: "Did someone or something in your life teach you to
have this desire?"
Reply: "My mom was never happy with her body."

Fourth question: "What's your belief about this desire?"
Reply: "If I look good, I will feel good. If I feel and look good, I will
fit in."

Fifth question: "Is there anything you did that you regret doing?"
Reply: "Yeah. I spent all day being anxious about my looks. I gave it a
lot of my energy all day so I probably put more pressure on myself
than I should have. I wasn't in a good state of mind when I started
to get ready for the party."

Sixth question: "What could you do differently next time?"
Reply: "When I feel the pain I will give myself ninety seconds to
breathe and invite God in."

Seventh and final question: "Is there anything you would like to
confess and repent of before we appear before the Judge and see
your offender?"
Reply: "I confess and repent of giving my body too much power and
attention."

Sidenote: If someone else was involved in this scenario, this would be
your time either to ask for forgiveness for any foul play on your part or
to forgive the person the enemy used to hurt you. Forgiveness given and
received enables you to stand blameless, with clean hands and a pure heart,
before the Judge. Remember, Satan is the enemy. Neither you nor the person who hurt you is the enemy.

The Holy Spirit: "No problem. You're forgiven and free. Way to go telling me what you know! Now let's go nail your enemy!"

With the help of your attorney, your offender has nothing on you. No surprises are coming your way. You're ready to face your enemy for his day in court.

As you walk into the courtroom, you take your seat next to your attorney, the Holy Spirit. You look to the jury box expecting to see chairs filled with peers, but all you see is Jesus. Just Jesus. He is the only One qualified to sit there because He is the only One who knows what it's like to be you—a human being who belongs to God in a broken world. His eyes crinkle and light up at the sight of you. His soft smile, which says, *I've got you*, fills you with comfort.

Suddenly, Satan, your enemy, walks in. He flashes a cocky smile as he shuffles forward with his hands and feet rattling in shackles. The sound of his chains is deafening. He takes his seat alone at the table adjacent to yours. He has no attorney. In his arrogance he thinks he's smart enough to represent himself. The words "All rise!" bellow through the room. In walks the honorable Judge: God, your Father in heaven. His robe commands authority and respect. In His presence, you know this is an open-and-shut case.

Satan takes the witness stand. There's no need to swear anyone in because lies can't be spoken here. (It's like the movie *Liar, Liar* when Jim Carey's character, the perpetual liar Fletcher Reede, can no longer speak anything but the truth.)

The Holy Spirit cuts to the chase with His questioning: "When this incident occurred, what was your motive? What were you trying to do?"

Satan's response: "I was trying to kill, steal, and destroy your client. It's the only thing I know to do."

"Why do you want to harm my client?" your attorney asks.

"I am jealous. I want what she has. She has beauty. Not just on the outside but the inside too. She loves God and really likes Him too. I once had that. And since the Judge has told me I can never again have what she has, I and a legion of others who work for me do everything we can to distort

God's beauty on earth in hopes of making the things of this world look more like the place we come from—hell. We hope they will work with us to work against God. We can't stand Him. *Hate* isn't a strong enough word."

"Please explain the weapons you use to execute your plan."

"Temptation is our favorite weapon," Satan says. "We tempt people to want something, anything, more than God. For example, your client spends a lot of time wanting her body to change. Although I can't read her thoughts, she talks about it incessantly. She's an easy target.

"When people give into temptation, first comes pleasure, then comes our favorite part, pain. That becomes our entry point to shame and fear, our chance to confuse them so they believe what we say. As human beings, with bodies, living in a material world, they tend to put a lot of confidence in what they feel, hear, and see. If we can keep them focusing on that, we can keep them stuck in a cycle of wanting pleasures that bring more pain. And people in pain help us do destructive things, since as you can see, I can't use my hands," he continues, rattling the handcuffs behind his back.

The Judge has heard enough.

"Satan, shame on you. I continue to find your crimes against humanity heinous and insidious. When will you learn? You will never have any part of Me, My children, or My Kingdom. Your acts will never prevail against My plans or My people, including this one-of-a-kind beautiful child of Mine right in front of Me.

"Satan, you are a murderer, a liar, and a thief. Nothing good or redemptive is in you."

The Judge motions for Satan to look at the jury box where Jesus sits. The Judge asks Jesus for a decision. Without hesitation, Jesus looks at Satan and says firmly, "Guilty."

The Judge declares, "By the blood of and in the name of My Son, Jesus, I sentence you and the lies you speak to go back to hell for eternity. You shall remain in your chains! The court is adjourned."

Bang! The gavel drops.

As he is swept away immediately in his rattling chains, the look of fury on Satan's face conveys a message. He should never have messed with you.

The Holy Spirit sweeps you up in a dance of delight and shouts,

"Together, we just destroyed Satan's plans! Let's do that all the time!" The Judge rushes down from His box as Jesus makes a beeline toward you. Tucked inside this circle of joy, your body feels like home. You feel courageous, warm, safe, and free.

Metabolize

Mind

Take another destructive thought about your body and put it on trial. You begin by having your private meeting with your attorney, the Holy Spirit. Together you make a plan for a successful trial where the enemy is condemned, not you! Work through the following questions in order to prepare.

- When the negative thought came, what were you desiring?
- What makes acquiring what you desire so difficult?
- Did something or someone in your life teach you to have that desire?
- What's your belief about this desire?
- Is there anything you did that you regret doing?
- What would you like to do differently next time?
- Is there anything you need to ask or extend forgiveness for?

Next, play out the remainder of the court scene where the enemy is forced to stop lying and tell the truth, and receives his sentencing back to hell. Be sure to take a moment to celebrate the victory in a joyful dance with your Father, Jesus, and the Holy Spirit.

Mouth

God, save me from the busyness of mind that keeps me from taking thoughts captive and putting them under eternal lock and key. Help me make my thoughts obedient to Your Word. I employ You, Holy Spirit, as my Advocate to argue my case before my enemies so I may continue to live free in my Father's Kingdom. Help me be about my Father's business and not my busyness. Help me have the mind of Christ. Amen.

Move

Take ten minutes to listen to this Be Still and Be Loved meditation that goes along with what you just read: https://www.revelationwellness.org/tbr/still/. Sometime today, lace up your shoes and go for twenty minutes of movement while listening to this audio recording: https://www.revelation wellness.org/tbr/move/.

Taking Ownership

And he said to him, "Son, you are always
with me, and all that is mine is yours."

LUKE 15:31

CHAPTER 21

DON'T LOSE THE KEYS

FOR YEARS MY MOM WAS EMPLOYED by the local school system. She loved working with children. She was a child herself in many ways, holding on to the innocence of a childhood she never had a chance to live. Without a college degree, she couldn't officially teach. Instead, she took the second-best role, getting paid minimum wage as a teacher's aide. Teachers *l-o-v-e-d* my mom. She was known for going over and beyond her role as an aide, whether cleaning desks, organizing closets, filing worksheets, wiping noses, or even taking recess duty for teachers wanting a break from the blazing Arizona sun. I never knew her to say no to any job.

Mom taught me that the most important person at school was not the principal but the janitor. The custodian, the one who cleans the toilets and mops the sweaty gym floor, has something nobody else in the school has: a ring filled with master keys to every room in the school. He can access the kitchen and its freezer filled with cookie dough and ice cream bars, as well as the office where cabinets are full of confidential student files.

Just as the school janitors' role gives them unfettered access to the school building, so our role as God's children comes with 24-7, 365-day access to God. We've been given keys, which give us power, and power belongs to those with authority.

Jesus is the Word made flesh (John 1:14). This means that when Jesus walked the earth, He knew the Word of God like the back of His hand. The scribes and the Pharisees, the religious leaders in Jesus' day, also knew the Word of God. From their youth, they'd studied and memorized it. But when Jesus showed up in their houses of worship and taught from the Scriptures, the people recognized that something profound had happened.

> On the Sabbath [Jesus] entered the synagogue and was teaching.
> And they were astonished at his teaching, for he taught them as
> one who had authority, and not as the scribes.
> MARK 1:21-22

When Jesus stood and spoke, He had something no other teacher had. He had authority. He didn't teach like a memory champion flexing his cognitive skills but like One who knew Scripture and had the power to back up what He was saying. As Jesus prepared His disciples for His execution, He assured them: "Heaven and earth will pass away, but my words will never pass away" (Matthew 24:35, NIV).

From the top of His head to the bottom of His feet, from the inside of His soul to the surface of His skin, Jesus believed in what He was saying. He could speak with authority because He was there when His Father spoke all that we see into existence. Jesus, sent by the Father to show the world God's Kingdom, spoke the words people needed to hear. Before Jesus came, they were all like sheep without a shepherd, wandering about trying to get their needs met. They needed a Good Shepherd to take authority over the wolves that tried to kill, steal, and destroy them; to protect and provide for them; and to lead them into pleasant places.

Knowledge of Scripture alone doesn't give us authority over our enemies; if it did, the scribes could have brought about world peace. Knowledge of Scripture alone doesn't have the power to bring about change. Only intimacy with our Creator, being known by God and coming to a deep knowing of Him, brings change.

---

*Only intimacy with our Creator, being known by God
and coming to a deep knowing of Him, brings change.*

Before I married my husband, I knew him as the blue-eyed British boy who always showed up early for my group fitness boxing class to help me hang the heavy bag. From our casual chats, I knew about some of his interests. But now, after twenty-five years of marriage, I really know my husband. I've spent more time with him than any other person on earth. I've loved him and been annoyed by him. And he really knows me—better than anyone else. We've gone through very joyful and sorrowful challenges together—trials that could have ruined us. But in the end, we've chosen to know and be known by each other over and over again. I know Simon, and I am known by Simon. God is looking for the same kind of commitment and intimacy from His people. He's looking for those who aren't in relationship to get something from Him (like some of the Pharisees who wanted prestige) but simply to be with Him. People who know God and His Word and are known by Him intimately, not just cognitively, are people God can trust with power and authority.

In the beginning, Jesus was with God (John 1:1). He has always existed with the Father. Other than that fateful moment when the Father had to turn His face from His Son because Jesus had taken the wrath for our sins upon Himself, there has never been a time when He hasn't been with His Father.

The Real Source of Authority

You know that rules cannot save you, because you've tried the workout programs and eating plans, and none of them seem to stick. Sure, in a moment of success, you may feel like you've got this thing nailed; you've got some authority over it. Memorizing and following rules gives us a false sense of authority. But then trouble comes and something knocks you off your feet. You don't need more rules to live by but a God to lead and shepherd you. In fact, you have a Good Shepherd. He loves to spend time with His sheep, to the point that they know His voice and do what He says:

My sheep listen to my voice; I know them, and they follow me. I give them eternal life, and they shall never perish; no one will snatch them out of my hand. My Father, who has given them to me, is greater than all; no one can snatch them out of my Father's hand. I and the Father are one.

JOHN 10:27-30, NIV

You don't need more rules to live by but
a God to lead and shepherd you.

Knowing and following God in this humble and intimate way—and having the courage to do what He says—is how we exercise our authority. This is how Jesus lived in His body.

Stephanie grew up in a Christian home and loved the Lord as far back as she could remember. She had no idea why God was nudging her to attend our Revelation Wellness instructor training because she had no desire to teach a fitness class. She had, however, struggled most of her life to feel good in her skin, especially when it came to being intimate with her husband. When she couldn't stop thinking about attending this unique discipleship training, Stephanie signed up. Her insecurity around her body had intensified a few years before when she discovered her husband's pornography addiction. He was actually relieved when his secret was no longer hidden because he finally felt able to get the help and treatment he needed. He loved Stephanie and their children and didn't want to lose his family. He was committed to his recovery. Stephanie wanted to believe him, but her already fragile body image felt shattered.

Now in training, Stephanie was learning how her physical body intersects with her faith. One day her small group got into a deep discussion about all the things that hindered them from living in freedom. "I wish I could be in my body and be free with my husband sexually. Is that even possible?" she asked the group.

To cap off the nine weeks of training, Stephanie took part in an instructor retreat. During the first night's worship, the group engaged in a time of healing prayer. Stephanie began to sense the Lord's nearness as she sought Him with others. *I won't quit on you until you are free, Stephanie*, she sensed God telling her. Every day of the retreat, He chipped away at Stephanie's guarded heart. On the night we focused on forgiveness, Stephanie had a vision of herself. She was standing naked before the Cross, feeling free and totally accepted by her Creator. "I know this sounds irreverent, Alisa, and a little crazy, but I can promise you, the image of me naked and unashamed, at the Cross, gave me back my authority. Jesus showed me that His sacrifice paid for me to have authority over my body and over my mind. My husband's sin is not about me. And my insecurities about my body are due to my being too focused on myself. I now know my assignment. I am going home to love my husband whom I love and choose and who is choosing me."

Stephanie has had her ups and downs since returning home, but she is more integrated than she's ever been. She and her husband continue to *work* on intimacy, knowing it's a choice to do so. She's heaven-bent on not quitting on the God who is healing her. Nor is she quitting on thoughts of loving-kindness toward her body and her husband, who is also choosing to be free.

Healthy authority occurs when we are absorbed in God's love and trust what He says. In the name of Jesus, and under His authority, we accept our freedom. We are free to love others and consider others better than ourselves. Someone else's win is not our loss, nor is someone else's loss our fault. In the Kingdom, there is no lack.

In Matthew 16, Jesus talks about the keys to His Kingdom.

Now when Jesus came into the district of Caesarea Philippi, he asked his disciples, "Who do people say that the Son of Man is?" And they said, "Some say John the Baptist, others say Elijah, and others Jeremiah or one of the prophets." He said to them, "But who do you say that I am?" Simon Peter replied, "You are the Christ, the Son of the living God." And Jesus answered him, "Blessed are you, Simon Bar-Jonah! For flesh and blood has not revealed this to you, but my Father who is in heaven. And I tell you, you are Peter, and on this rock I will build my church, and the gates of hell shall not prevail against it. I will give you the keys to the kingdom of heaven, and whatever you bind on earth shall be bound in heaven, and whatever you loose on earth shall be loosed in heaven."

MATTHEW 16:13-19

Notice three things that have happened for Peter (and us) to gain the keys to the Kingdom:

1. **He knew who God was personally in his heart, not just cognitively in his head.** Jesus asked Peter, "Who do *you* say that I am?" (emphasis mine). He didn't ask, "What does the Scripture say about Me?" Although knowing God's Word is powerful and absolutely necessary to living well, our authority comes from knowing the God whom Scripture is about.

2. **Peter told Jesus who He was, then Jesus told Peter who he was.** In response to Jesus' question about who He was, Peter said, "You are the Christ, the Son of the living God." Jesus, in turn, told Simon who he was: "And I tell you, *you are Peter*" (emphasis mine). The name *Peter* in Greek means "rock," and Jesus was acknowledging His disciple's role as an early confessor and leader of His church. In knowing who Jesus was, Peter knew who he was.

   If we want to know who we are, we must first know God.

3. **In knowing God personally and intimately, we gain the keys to the Kingdom of Heaven.** "*I will give you* the keys to the kingdom of heaven" (emphasis mine). Knowing who Jesus is makes it possible for us to truly know who we are. In this rightful knowing, we are given keys. With our keys, we have the power to bind and loose things on earth that will remain permanently bound or loosed in heaven.

   We have access to the heart of God, who gave our bodies form and called us by name to come home to Him. Just as the school janitor can enter any door, we hold the keys that provide us with access to the hidden things of heaven. We can bind the things that conflict with God's plan and loosen the things that agree with it.

When you look in the mirror and start to critique what you see, whether dimples on your thighs or lines on your face, pull out your keys and bind that line of thinking quickly! Kingdom citizens with Kingdom authority don't have time for *that*! Then with your key, loosen the blessings of God's love and truth over you and your circumstances. Unlike people with low self-esteem who feel like frauds for making positive statements to themselves, you will believe what you say when you and God are on intimate terms.

Our bodies are not what we worship. Our bodies are the place where worship occurs. So worship, friends, worship! When trouble comes, go for a walk, keeping Satan under your feet. Or when trouble comes, take a seat. Be still and breathe. God's forgiveness has made you free; now remain free by exercising your authority! Bind and loosen. Bind and loosen. Use your keys.

The old adage "Use it or lose it!" is true. It applies not only to our physical muscles and agility but to our spiritual authority. If we don't use the authority we have in Christ, it will shrivel up like a withered hand we never use. We mustn't forfeit our authority to an enemy who has every hope of building his hell-like kingdom on earth. But remember, your power doesn't come just from knowing God's truth but from knowing the God who backs up what He speaks.

We can't afford to let any thought, feeling, or choice we make in our bodies concerning our bodies steal our keys! We have good work to do with these bodies and the authority to do it. We are all janitors, heaven's cleanup crew responsible for taking out the trash!

As we cool down and move into the final stage of metabolizing our pain for our good, keep in mind that each stage of this workout builds upon the previous one. In the last section, stage 5, we considered how to stop living from the visible world and, through faith, live from God's unseen (for now) Kingdom. Our bodies are essential to making His Kingdom seen. We don't worship them, but we steward them well because they are part of God's original design for good on the earth.

At this point in exchanging our pain for health and freedom, we need to return to the Garden, to get back to God's original plan for making heaven seen through us. In the beginning, God, the One with ultimate authority over all creation, made us in His image. He breathed life into our nostrils, blessed us, and called us good. In our goodness (a state of being), we are to fill the earth with more good (a state of doing). To do good, we need two things: the ability to subdue the earth and the power to have dominion. Only Christ followers have been given the authority to fulfill God's original intention for us.

Every time we take an unhealthy thought captive, and when necessary, put it on trial, we make it obedient to God's original design for good. We put chaos into handcuffs and make it obedient to God's plan for peace. We exercise dominion and remind the enemy that the Cross sentenced him to eternal hell. He's trash, and he must go back to hell and burn in his eternal dumpster fire of lies.

Next time your enemy accuses you or uses someone to hurt you, be a good janitor by using your key and taking out the trash. Satan wants you to be harder on yourself through shaming, bingeing, restricting, or overworking. Don't let him trash-talk you. Remember that you are God's good idea! You have the authority to ensure that your body home is a fresh, clean, and inviting space for the Holy Spirit.

Keep growing in intimacy with God and use your keys!

Metabolize

Mind

1. How is the authority of Jesus different from the authority of men?
2. Who do you say Jesus is? Who does He say you are? And what has Jesus given you authority over when it comes to your physical health?
3. What would more intimacy with God mean for you?

Mouth

Father God, help me receive and exercise the authority You've given me over all creation. Come and heal my heart and mind from the hurts that distort the way I view and use authority. With a crown on my head and keys in my hand, I want to walk upright on the earth as a representative of Your Kingdom. Teach me how to have more intimacy with You, not just knowledge about You, so I may operate in the full authority You've given me. Come integrate my love for You with my knowledge about You. Amen.

Move

The easiest way to begin to grow in intimacy with God is to invite Him into every part of your life. That is the purpose of the Move section in each chapter. Every time you use a link provided in this section, you are getting physical with the God who created you. You are moving your body to be *with* Him and to hear from Him. To grow your soul and heal your body-mind pain, please keep pressing play on these links. Your intimacy with God is growing as you move your body, not just your heart and mind, closer to His! Let intimacy overflow into all areas of your life, into all the places God wants to be.

Take ten minutes to listen to this Be Still and Be Loved meditation that goes along with what you just read: https://www.revelationwellness.org /tbr/still/. Then sometime today, lace up your shoes and move for twenty minutes while listening to this link: https://www.revelationwellness.org/tbr /move/. Or try any other way to move your body with the movement links on page 274.

CHAPTER 22

HAVE A VISION
FOR YOUR FUTURE

GROWING UP, I lived in the biggest house on the block. Our house was obnoxiously large compared to the other two-bedroom homes in our neighborhood that had been built during the post–World War II boom. We weren't wealthy by any means, but my father liked to play rich and got a sense of accomplishment by giving my mom a home she could be proud of. Our house was always under some sort of construction. In five years, in fact, it doubled in size. I remember regularly seeing blueprints, like maps to a pirate's buried cache, rolled out on our kitchen table. And her home was my mom's treasure. Perhaps by using it as a canvas on which to create outer beauty, she was trying to control her inner chaos and lack of peace.

As God's image bearers, we all can create beauty. We need just two things: desire and vision. Desires can either help or hurt the working order and the beauty of our bodies, minds, and souls. Longing for anything more than God may help us survive, but it will never enable us to grow and build our lives as He intended. Ultimately, seeking peace in other people or things will lead only to frustration and crooked vision. For example, my mom longed for my dad to love and protect her body, but she never received that from him. I watched as she transferred those desires toward a vision of keeping order and beauty in her home.

I had a different vision. Rather than desiring a beautiful house, I worked for a beautiful body, a sort of mobile home to go with me wherever I went. If I looked good, I was sure I'd gain attention and respect. Before long, it was clear that my vision would get me no closer to lasting joy and peace than my mom's vision did for her. Mom's house eventually became dated and worn and had to be spruced up again. In my case, my body would get injured, and there was nothing I could do to prevent my body from aging.

I learned there is a better way. Conforming our desires to God's creates godly desires in us. That leads to a vision for the things we can build and the people we can be built into, so that heaven is seen on earth.

For lasting freedom in the way we feel, think, and act in our bodies, we must pay attention to our desires and our vision. One goes with the other. Desire motivates us to go after what we want, and our attention and energy go wherever we set our eyes. When the Israelites stopped desiring God above other things, the Lord spoke to the prophet Habakkuk, asking him to record what was to come for His people.

> And the LORD answered me: "Write the vision; make it plain on tablets, so he may run who reads it. For still the vision awaits its appointed time; it hastens to the end—it will not lie. If it seems slow, wait for it; it will surely come; it will not delay. Behold, his soul is puffed up; it is not upright within him, but the righteous shall live by his faith."
>
> HABAKKUK 2:2-4

The people of Judah were headed for captivity in Babylon, a ruthless and evil empire filled with licentiousness and iniquity. God wanted Habakkuk to share this vision of what was to come, even though it was not a good one. Why would God ask Habakkuk to deliver a terrible vision? The souls of God's people were puffed up and no longer upright. They thought they had a better plan for their lives than God's. They were no longer living by faith but for their flesh even though, as God told Habakkuk, "the righteous shall live by faith."

God's word to Habakkuk was not His original vision for His people. As we've seen, God created humans to co-reign and rule over creation. But when Adam and Eve gave in to Satan's temptation, sin entered the world. All things fractured, including our vision. Instead of having eyes solely for God, our eyes were opened to the knowledge of good and evil (Genesis 3:7). We now know and see things we weren't supposed to see and know. And since we aren't God, we see them crookedly. East of Eden, we all live with the ophthalmic spiritual disease of fractured vision.

We don't see our bodies correctly.

We don't see goodness correctly.

We don't see God correctly.

We Don't See Our Bodies Correctly

As a fitness instructor, I'm well aware of the difference between the way we experience our bodies and the way we see our bodies. Body schema refers to our awareness of our bodies—the way our brains connect to our bodies through sensory experience and motor skill. Our body schema helps us control our posture and movement. It's essential for us to complete any physical task, such as taking out the trash. People with cerebral palsy have a disrupted body schema. They don't receive the same sensory and motor input as those without this disorder. That can make a simple task, like filling a glass with water, challenging.

On the other hand, body image is the way we view our bodies in relationship to ourselves and the world around us. While body schema is mechanical and fact-based, body image is psychological and a matter of opinion.

The way we think and feel about our bodies affects the vision we have of ourselves and our assumptions about what others think when they see us. Just as a malfunctioning body schema could prevent us from riding a bike, a broken body image may make it challenging to take part in a family portrait or attend a social gathering.

As I write this chapter, we have lived through the second year of the global pandemic COVID-19. I have never been in more online meetings than I have in the past eighteen months. The other day, after hour four of back-to-back calls, it occurred to me that although video conferencing has been a gift during this season, too much of seeing ourselves as others see us can't be good for our brains. When we meet with someone in person, we don't see them seeing us. We only see them. That's the way being with others is supposed to be. God didn't give us a body to enter a room with either a "Here I am!" boastful, look-at-me spirit or a "Wish I could disappear" shame-filled one. Like Jesus, we are to enter a room with an "Oh, there you are!" encouraging spirit. Our bodies weren't given to us so we could serve ourselves, but so we could love God and others. Too much focus on ourselves distorts our Kingdom vision.

I saw a meme go around social media some time ago, and whenever I recognize that I'm focusing on my body too much, I remember what it said: "Mother Teresa didn't have time to sit around and worry about the shape of her biceps. She had crud to do" (though *crud* wasn't the actual four-letter word used). In other words, Mother Teresa didn't let her body image get in the way of her body schema.

When we focus on ourselves too much, we lose sight of our role as image bearers of God.

We Don't See Goodness Correctly

Because of sin we have no problem seeing problems. Allow me to give you an example of what this looks like.

Scenario: You enjoy your job, and you do good work. Your boss says he would like to meet with you on Monday. Which of the following conclusions do you immediately come to?

a. *Shoot. I guess I'm not doing my job as well as I thought I was, and my boss probably wants to talk to me about my work. What if he demotes me or, even worse, fires me? I better start coming up with my plan B.*

b. *Wow! This is great! I'm looking forward to some face-to-face time with the boss. Perhaps he wants to give me kudos in person, or a promotion, or maybe even a raise! Wow! I am really looking forward to Monday!*

I know choice b seems wildly optimistic compared to the painful realities we've encountered in survival mode, but we are now citizens of God's Kingdom. And scenario b should be our default possibility when we show up to the places we live, work, study, and play with a vision for how we can represent God's Kingdom. We must keep our minds set on the Kingdom and our eyes filled with Kingdom vision. Being grateful for a good job and our good bodies, which give us the ability to do good work, is one way we can make the vision of God's unseen Kingdom seen.

Jesus came to earth and experienced physical, mental, and emotional pain in His body while continuing to think, feel, and choose in line with His vision of His Father's goodness. Even now, people who think good thoughts and maintain their Father's good vision have the ability to create more good all around them.

People who think good thoughts and maintain their Father's good vision have the ability to create more good all around them.

We Don't See God Correctly

Our eyes can look at only one thing at any time. If my right eye looks left and my left eye looks right, my eyes will cross. I won't see clearly or correctly. When sin entered the world, our eyes got crossed, and we stopped seeing God correctly. But when Jesus came to earth to redeem mankind, He did so with clear vision. He didn't waver when the Jewish leaders accused Him of blasphemy and wrongdoing because He healed on the Sabbath. He told them, "Truly, truly, I say to you, the Son can do nothing of his own accord, but only what he sees the Father doing. For whatever the Father does, that the Son does likewise" (John 5:19-20).

Jesus came to earth with a single vision: to do His Father's will in His physical body. In fact, He said He could do nothing of His own accord. Think about that! When Jesus uses the word *only*, He acknowledges a limitation placed on the use of His power. Jesus knew that effectiveness came from doing only what He saw His Father doing. Jesus lived in a noisy world filled with needy people, with a body that ached, with sore feet and a broken heart. Yet He knew that if He didn't keep His full attention on His Father, He couldn't do anything.

We, too, can take what hurts us in our earthly bodies and do bigger things than simply trying for smaller jeans and bigger muscles, but that requires us to keep our eyes on what our Father is doing. He never runs out of options and possibilities. To accomplish lasting results for God's Kingdom, we must keep our eyes on the One from whom our help comes. Where our attention goes, the power flows.

Where our attention goes, the power flows.

A study conducted at the University of Chicago by Dr. Judd Biasiotto demonstrated the power of visualization. A random group of students were asked to make basketball free throws. The students took their best shots, and their scores were tallied. Next the students were broken up into three groups. One group was told not to touch a basketball for thirty days. Another practiced free throws an hour a day for thirty days. The final group was asked to come to the gym for thirty days to visualize themselves making free throws. After that month, the groups were asked to come back and make their free throw shots again. As you can imagine, the group that didn't touch a basketball showed no improvement. The group that practiced every day showed a 24 percent increase in successful free throws. Now get this: The group that simply sat in the gym and visualized themselves making the shots showed a 23 percent improvement in successful attempts—only one percent less than the group that did the very thing they were visualizing.[1]

Now that you've read about this study, you may be thinking, *Great, Alisa. All I need to do is visualize myself living well in my body. I'll just do that. I'll save myself all the other work.* To that, I say, not so fast. First, remember that this book is designed to help us learn to transform the pain we've lived through in our bodies and brains so that it serves the greater purposes of God. Having a purpose is useless if we don't act on it. The people in the group who only visualized making free throws eventually returned to the free throw line to take their shots and demonstrate how much they'd improved. We can't just sit back and have a vision of living well and free in our body. We must act according to the vision God gives us. As we pursue God's deeper healing love and have eyes for Him only (not the shape of our waistlines), we will overflow with the energy we need to take our shots; to think, feel, and choose according to God's will. Like Jesus, we must keep God's vision in our sights *and* actually live it out.

Imagine the improvement a fourth group would have made in Dr. Biasiotto's study—one that practiced both the skills of visualizing free throws and actually shooting the free throws. Likewise, we must remain focused on the Father's vision for us *and* do His will as Jesus did.

> Let us fix our eyes on Jesus, the author and perfecter of our faith,
> who for the joy set before him endured the cross, scorning its
> shame, and sat down at the right hand of the throne of God.
> HEBREWS 12:1-2, NIV

As we live this way, it will be harder for us to go against His will. Choices that could harm our mental and physical health and immunity will become less attractive. We won't try to keep our eyes on two opposing goals (e.g., the shape of our thighs and the growth of God's Kingdom).

It's time to stop entertaining the world's ideas of what your body is meant to look like and do. With your mind on Christ and the life He lived in His body, keep your eyes on the Father. Ask Him to give you His vision. Keep that vision before you and take your shot!

Metabolize

Mind

Get quiet for a moment. Take a few deep breaths, inhaling for a count of four and then exhaling for a count of four. Then ask the Holy Spirit to help answer this prayer:

Father, show me what You want to do when it comes to my body schema (ability) and body image (psychology).

Write down everything you hear and see in your journal. Try to be as specific as possible and invite all your senses (sound, smell, touch, and taste) into God's vision.

Then draw like nobody is watching! Do your best to turn the words God spoke into some sort of picture or image. Once complete, keep that image in your phone, on the fridge, or anywhere you can look when you are tempted to question your body's worth and ability.

Sidenote: TIP (Think in Pictures). That's how memory champions remember abstract concepts at length. When you read God's Word, ask the Holy Spirit to help you TIP.

Here's an example of TIP: You read "For God gave us a spirit not of fear but of power and love and self-control" (2 Timothy 1:7). Use your creativity (which we all have, even if some art teacher told you that you didn't). Take a moment to close your eyes and imagine the verse playing out in the theater of your mind. Perhaps you see yourself standing in the corner of a room, filled with people, hiding and feeling insecure about your body. Next, see the kind face of Jesus noticing you. He walks over and removes a heavy black cloak (or whatever represents fear and timidity to you) from your shoulders. Then watch Jesus reach inside His robe for an orb of light (power) to place on your chest. This light jump-starts your heart and fills you with warmth (love). Your cheeks flush with a healthy pink glow as the bright light shoots up your chest cavity until it reaches your head. Suddenly you can think like a responder, not a reactor, which enables you to feel you belong here, knowing you aren't here for yourself but with God to represent God (self-control).

I know this exercise may feel weird, but trust me when I say that it will allow the Word to become more personal and intimate for you. When Jesus taught the people using parables, they naturally visualized the stories in pictures, which can be a powerful way for the love of God to use our minds to reach our hearts as well.

Mouth

God, bind my flesh and be my vision. In Jesus' name, Amen.

Move

Take ten minutes to listen to this Be Still and Be Loved meditation: https://www.revelationwellness.org/tbr/still/. Sometime today, lace up your shoes and go for twenty minutes of movement while listening to this audio recording: https://www.revelationwellness.org/tbr/move/.

CHAPTER 23

WORDS CREATE YOUR WORLD

"One day your mouth is going to get you into big trouble."

Allison recalls her mom and dad telling her this often as she was growing up. Her parents were Christian fundamentalists who judged people on what they did. Though Allison's parents didn't always act on their own beliefs, they expected her to do whatever they said. This didn't sit well with Allison's heart for justice. When she didn't agree with someone, she was quick to let that person know. So when her parents grounded her for talking back, guess what she did? Yup. She talked (or more like yelled) back again. When grounded, Allison had a knack for turning one week of punishment into two.

One day as she sulked in her bedroom jail cell at the start of a one-month sentence, her older brother walked in. She was still trying to catch her breath and wipe away her tears when he hugged her. Then he said, "Hey, Ali. When Mom and Dad say or do something you don't agree with, don't talk back. Just do what I do and take it. Your words are only fueling their anger and making the outcome worse for you."

Allison knew her brother was right in one sense, but he was also a pro at suppressing his feelings. At least Allison received a payoff by releasing her fury. She was convinced that something that felt so good in the moment had to make some movement toward change, albeit usually just an increase in the time she was imprisoned in her bedroom. Allison's brain wasn't fully developed, and she was living in a house of pain. Her brain's drug of choice to cope with that pain was to shout hateful words.

Now years later, not only was Allison older, but she hated her body because of her weight. She felt plagued by condemning thoughts that turned into negative words about her body. She was stuck in a destructive habit loop. Worse yet, she knew her eight-year-old daughter watched her weigh herself and speak negatively about her body. Allison desperately wanted to love and accept her body, if only for her daughter's sake.

The Weight of Words

Words are great allies to our pain—battle buddies with swords and explosives, willing to charge the front line in the war for our hearts. Take a moment to think about the words you have thought or said about your body. (Go ahead . . . take a moment. Without fear. Take a breath and think.)

I would bet my last dollar that the words that first came to your mind are negative and outnumber the positive ones. We've heard that words can't break our bones like sticks and stones can, but one thing is for sure—negative words *stick*! And sin makes it challenging to receive kind words. They slide off us like a fried egg in a Teflon pan, while negative words stick like flies in glue. The stickiness of painful words isn't your fault; it's one effect of living in a fallen world with a brain that is just trying to keep you alive and surviving.

Our brains are more likely to remember negative words and experiences so we can adjust our choices and avoid future pain. Negative and fearful words often rise up during our fight, flight, or freeze response. When we unleash them, they can help us release stress and anxiety. (This is why people tend to feel better after they've screamed or talked back to someone.) Remember, our brains naturally want to conserve energy and are risk averse. That is why we don't naturally seek out adverse moments that interrupt our safety or our status quo, unless we choose to challenge the construct of comfort we find ourselves in.

For optimal brain and body health, we must let God's Word have first and final say. In the middle place, between first and final say, we are invited to come to God with our words. And by the way, it's not a sin to cry, shout, or scream in the presence of God so we can release stress and anxiety. His lap is big enough for our pain, and His heart can handle the words we say. When my kids were little and were harassed by a bully on the playground, they ran to me in hysterics. I would hug them and do my best to calm them down. Then I'd gently ask, "What's wrong? Use your words." In the same way, God wants us to run to Him, using words to express our pain. He wants to hear our words, even if they are wrong. If we stay long enough in His presence, He will tell us what is true—the right words to think and say.

For optimal brain and body health,
we must let God's Word have first and final say.

No one taught me how to go to God with my pain. Like Allison, I learned to talk back to people instead of talking to God. When God gets the first and final say, there will be times He asks us to do things that make us afraid, like forgiving the person who did something wrong or said hurtful things.

Words have power! Words are thoughts with muscle. Words can build up or take down. And words don't have to be spoken to deliver a knockout punch.

Masaru Emoto, a Japanese businessman and pseudoscientist, claimed that exposure to words could affect the molecular structure of water. He exposed water in glasses to various words, pictures, and music. He placed words and phrases like *I hate you* and *fear* as well as *I love you* and *peace* on glasses of water. He then froze the water and, via microscopic photography, studied the structure of the ice crystals. Dr. Emoto found that water with the positive words created visually pleasing ice crystals, while negative words created ugly ice formations. He reported that when water was exposed to pleasing music, it created beautiful crystals, while the distorted sounds of heavy metal led to dull ice crystals.[1] Because Emoto was not a scientist and declined to reproduce the experiment under scientific testing criteria, his study is considered unreliable. Even if Emoto's study was fringe science, we can all agree that negative thoughts clamoring around in our minds don't make us feel more beautiful and strong, nor do they make us stand taller. Instead, negative words distort our brain and body image. A poor thought or poorly spoken word can cause us to slump our shoulders, bury our chins, and gaze down at our feet. Negative words said about us tend to make us more self-conscious and self-absorbed. The more focused we become on ourselves, the less fellowship we have with God. Do you know anyone who feels more open-hearted, connected, and trusting of God when a negative word is spoken? Probably not. God corrects us, yes. But when He does, He doesn't condemn us or speak harshly to us. His words express His love and add beauty; they don't take it away.

Negative words come from our enemy who wants to steal, kill, and destroy our lives. Whenever Satan spots a slight crack or crevice of separation between God and us, he will sneak in and try taking us captive. We must constantly take out the trash of his negative thoughts if we want our bodies and brains to stay well and free.

Words Create Worlds

When he was very little, my son, Jack, had a picture book made of cardboard that was filled with pictures of colorful objects and the word that went with each item. Jack's first and favorite word in that book was *ball*, or as he said, "Bawwwwwl." Jack's tiny tongue muscle did its very best to form the sound of the *l*.

When he was able to match the right word to that picture, I rejoiced with an outburst and a big mama hug. Why? Because my son was beginning to make sense of the world around him and use his words appropriately. He had matched the image to the correct word.

We all could use this type of retraining for our bodies and brains. We need to match our image-bearing bodies to the Word that was in the beginning. When we match who we are with the image of the God who made us and called us "very good" (Genesis 1:31), we fill our being with the goodness of God. Our bodies become vessels for containing the thoughts of God and vehicles for delivering the words God wants to say.

Words create our world. They help us define what we see. When you were a child, someone in authority helped you find the words to describe what you saw or wanted. That perspective molded your long-term worldview. Whether you see a world filled with wonder or a world at war has much to do with the one who taught you how to speak. But as followers of Christ, your citizenship has been transferred from this world to His Kingdom. God, your Father, now teaches you how to speak. The question that remains is this: From which domain will you think and find your words? From the Kingdom of our Father or the kingdom of this world?

All of God's goodness became visible with these words: "And God said . . ." (Genesis 1:3, 6, 9, 11, 14, 20, 24, 26, 28, 29). A good God made unseen things seen through the power of His words. They brought forth the highpoint of His creation, Adam and Eve. Blessed by God, they were told to increase good while subduing the earth and having dominion. Remember, subduing and having dominion are terms denoting power and strength. But God didn't hand us weapons like sticks and stones to break our enemy's bones in our quest to subdue and have dominion. He handed us His own tools—words.

As Adam's first good work, God didn't ask him to exert physical strength by taking his body for a test run. The Lord didn't check to see if Adam's glutes, hamstrings, and quadriceps were strong enough to flip a tire or uproot a tree. He didn't test Adam's endurance or the oxygen uptake of Adam's lungs, asking him to sprint. No, rather than putting Adam's body to the test during his first task in the Garden, God put his mind to work. Adam spent his first day on the job of adding good and having dominion by speaking—naming all the living creatures:

> Now out of the ground the LORD God had formed every beast of
> the field and every bird of the heavens and brought them to the
> man to see what he would call them. And whatever the man called
> every living creature, that was its name.
>
> GENESIS 2:19

Adam's first work was to imitate God by using the same weapon and power tool for building heaven on earth that He had used—words.

Like a skilled carpenter with a table saw or a soldier training for war, we must learn to use our words like tools and weapons. We don't want to saw off our fingers when confused by the smoke bomb of pain the enemy throws our way or be the cause of friendly fire, mistakenly aiming our weapon at someone we love.

I am pretty sure Jesus' brother James would have made a great personal trainer. He seems to have been a man of action. He is the one who said that our faith is nothing if we don't have good works to prove it (James 2:17). He also gives us one of the greatest passages in Scripture about our tongue, along with guidance on how we are to train it:

> We all stumble in many ways. And if anyone does not stumble in what he says, he is a perfect man, able also to bridle his whole body. If we put bits into the mouths of horses so that they obey us, we guide their whole bodies as well. Look at the ships also: though they are so large and are driven by strong winds, they are guided by a very small rudder wherever the will of the pilot directs. So also the tongue is a small member, yet it boasts of great things. How great a forest is set ablaze by such a small fire! And the tongue is a fire, a world of unrighteousness. The tongue is set among our members, staining the whole body, setting on fire the entire course of life, and set on fire by hell.
>
> JAMES 3:2-6

Look how powerful something so small can be! Our tongues can:

- keep our body from sin
- guide us into thinking, feeling, and doing the right thing
- make great boasts
- break our relationship with God
- damage our body's health
- destroy our entire life

The Bible is clear: The words we speak with our tongues affect the outcome of our lives. With our words we can either build things up or tear things down, including the health of our brains and our immune systems.

In their book *Words Can Change Your Brain*, Andrew Newberg and Mark Robert Waldman say, "The more you stay focused on negative words and thoughts, the more you can actually damage key structures that regulate your memory, feelings, and emotions. You may disrupt your sleep, your appetite, and the way your brain regulates happiness, longevity, and health."[2]

Newberg and Waldman back up what God has already said about the power of words. The following verses are from Proverbs, a wisdom book of the Bible. Notice how these verses connect the use of words to the needs of our bodies and the misplaced desires that cause us pain.

> Gentle words are a tree of life;
> a deceitful tongue crushes the spirit.
> PROVERBS 15:4, NLT

> Kind words are like honey—
> sweet to the soul and healthy for the body.
> PROVERBS 16:24, NLT

Key point: Kind words spoken about our bodies lead to good health.

> Wise words are like deep waters;
> wisdom flows from the wise like a bubbling brook.
> PROVERBS 18:4, NLT

Key point: Good words hydrate thirsty souls who thought better bodies would quench their thirst.

> Wise words satisfy like a good meal;
> the right words bring satisfaction.
> PROVERBS 18:20, NLT

Key point: Good words feed hungry souls who thought better bodies would satisfy their hunger.

> Death and life are in the power of the tongue,
> and those who love it will eat its fruits.
> PROVERBS 18:21

Key point: If we speak life, we will eat and be satisfied. If we speak poorly, we will live hungry.

The words we use provide the energy for metabolizing our pain. We can train ourselves to use life-giving words to reap more life. If we use life-stealing words instead, we will lack the energy we need to work through our pain. We may survive and even stay safe using hurtful words, but only when we open our hearts can we fill our mouths with words that bring change.

Before you get to work toning your body, train your tongue. If you begin paying attention to the words you say, you will discover the deceptions hidden in your heart and mind: "For the mouth speaks what the heart is full of" (Luke 6:45, NIV).

Before you get to work toning your body, train your tongue.

Your body can be any size you want it to be as long as you cultivate the heart God wants you to have. Out of your heart, your mouth speaks!

Metabolize

Mind

1. How often do you think or say unkind things about your body?
2. Pick one of the proverbs about our bodies and our health (see pages 253–254). Now TIP it! Think in pictures by drawing out the verse on a piece of paper. Once finished, consider putting that picture somewhere you need to see it to remember it.

3. Ask the Holy Spirit to show you a picture of what negative words do to you and what kind words do to you. Then describe or draw those images.

Mouth

God, help me think and say the words You are saying. Amen.

Move

If you have a hard time being kind with your words, you need a clearer vision of God's grace. The two practices below will help improve your self-talk.

- **Slow is kind.** Kind words come more easily to those who are calm in the Spirit. To prepare your mind for action the next time you are in pain, slow down your speech and be deliberate with what you say. Pay attention to the words you choose and speak. Notice how your words feel on the tip of your tongue, how they squeeze through your teeth, and how the muscles of your mouth move to make sounds. Speak crisply and clearly. Language is truly a gift—an instrument to practice and to play. Get curious about how you're using it!

- **Take inventory.** This is a humbling exercise. Spend twenty-four hours taking inventory of the words you say. Place a three-by-five card or any small piece of paper in your purse or pocket. Every time you notice yourself thinking or saying negative words, rip a portion of the card and throw it away. Then make a hash mark in the middle of the paper to account for the word you thought or said. At the end of the day, see how big or small your paper is and how often you used harsh words toward yourself or another. Reflect on your day with curiosity and without judgment. We can't change what we don't recognize, and God helps the humble.

Take ten minutes to listen to this Be Still and Be Loved meditation on the kindness of God and His words: https://www.revelationwellness.org/tbr/still/. Then sometime today, move your body kindly while listening to this audio recording: https://www.revelationwellness.org/tbr/move/.

CHAPTER 24

CELEBRATE!

Tammy gets off the bus with a look of fear and trepidation in her eyes. Mountains surround her, and the smell of pine trees fills the air. After nine hours of travel, she just wants to get off the bus and quickly find her room. For over two months, she has been taking part in Revelation Wellness instructor training, watching herself transform from the inside out as she embraces freedom for herself and learns how to set others free too. Now that she's arrived for the five-day intensive retreat, she wonders what she's gotten herself into. No one else she knows is registered for the event. Surrounded by two hundred men and women in athletic leisurewear, Tammy is greeted by Revelation Wellness staffers and instructors holding up and waving cardboard signs bearing messages like "There you are!" "You are a good idea!" and "You belong here!"

Goodness, these people are kind of annoyingly happy, she thinks. The moment is almost too much to take in. Tammy's eyes dart through the celebratory crowd, looking for at least one familiar face. She finally relaxes when she spots her small group leader.

Tammy has brought a lot of her insecurities with her to this retreat. She thinks she looks nothing like the other fitness influencers on Instagram. The few workout clothes she owns are last year's styles, which she picked up from the clearance section at Old Navy. Not only has she not lost an ounce of her "baby weight," but she has gained several pounds since giving birth for the final time six years ago. In fact, she's still scratching her head, wondering why the Lord would call her to a faith and fitness ministry. She's never loved exercise or weekly meal prep. Taking care of her body feels more like a burden, her cross to bear. But the Lord kept tugging at Tammy's heart, and she wanted to be obedient to the gentle nudge of the Spirit that kept telling her, *Come*. Now she is committed to learning what she needs to know to reconnect to God and use her body as a tool to spread the gospel.

The Lord wants to celebrate Tammy. He wants her to know that she is His beloved daughter with whom He is well pleased. He saw her unformed body in her mother's womb, the same body she is prone to criticize. God has good plans for her, and He knows the reason she feels stuck in her life and with her body, thinking and talking negatively. It's time for her to be a doer of God's Word and not just a hearer. Over the next five days, she will use her body to speak and do. She will do and say things she *never* thought possible. Tammy is about to experience physical and spiritual neuroplasticity—a rewiring of her brain as she brings her body before God to renew all of her—heart, soul, and mind.

As we come to these final moments of our workout together, I wish I could tell you that you will no longer have to deal with the pain that can get stuck in your body and negatively affect your brain. Helping you avoid pain was never the goal of this book. As Paul says, "To live is Christ and to die is gain" (Philippians 1:21). While we live on this earth, we are to live like Christ. That means we will experience pain and suffering, like He did. Living like Christ will at times feel like dying as we put to death desires that are not God's. The good news for our bodies is this: We have the Holy Spirit, the presence of God in us, to help us endure and remind us of the coming day when we will experience no more pain.

With our workout coming to an end, you may wonder how to know if you're processing your pain well and whether you're staying free. If so, ask yourself this question: *How's my joy?*

Joy is the energy of heaven that enabled Jesus to endure His pain and suffering: "For the joy set before him he endured the cross" (Hebrews 12:2, NIV).

And if you want to know what's happening in heaven right now, look to Romans 14:17: "For the kingdom of God is not a matter of eating and drinking, but of righteousness, peace and joy in the Holy Spirit" (Romans 14:17, NIV).

Heaven is full of joy right now. Our great cloud of witnesses of faith are not busy counting calories, drinking protein shakes, or wondering what to eat in their heavenly home. They are full of joy. They are bubbling up and overflowing with joy. They are celebrating and enjoying the Lord! As God's children who belong to His Kingdom, we can do here and now what our family is doing there—celebrate God's victory!

Joy is not happiness. Happiness is attached to circumstances that come and go, such as a number on a scale. Happiness is temporal, while joy is eternal. Happiness is earthbound while joy is heaven sent. Joy is our confidence that, on the Cross, God put to death everything that tries to kill, steal, and destroy us. Joy is confidence that God is good no matter our circumstances. Joy is confidence in God—or what I like to call Godfidence. People with joy can lose their job, loved ones, or health and grieve without losing hope in God. Like the apostle Paul says, joyful people can say

> I know what it is to be in need, and I know what it is to have
> plenty. I have learned the secret of being content in any and every
> situation, whether well fed or hungry, whether living in plenty or
> in want. I can do all this through him who gives me strength.
>
> PHILIPPIANS 4:12-13, NIV

Paul's "secret" to contentment was joy. And since joy comes from God, the joy of the Lord was Paul's strength. He had taken to heart the Old Testament prophet Nehemiah's declaration: "Do not be grieved, for the joy of the Lord is your strength" (Nehemiah 8:10).

The joy of the Lord is the strongest of strengths. The joy of the Lord surpasses our understanding of what it means to be strong. The Lord is not opposed to us lifting weights to gain bodily strength or challenging our learning to build mental strength, but all our strength gains pale in comparison to the strength of God's joy. Joy transcends all earthly power and makes it possible for God's people to share in Christ's victory, even when they're suffering.

The Lord is not opposed to us lifting weights,
but our strength gains pale in comparison
to the strength of God's joy.

When we have the joy of the Lord, we have confidence that God will make a way, regardless of our circumstances. Just as the cross Jesus bore made God's Good News available to all, people with joy believe God will put their pain to good use. When we have the joy of the Lord, there is nothing we can't endure.

When you feel your limbic (or emoting) brain signaling pain, lift the thought of Jesus up to the prefrontal cortex (or thinking) area of your brain. As you keep your mind set on Jesus, your body and mind will set themselves on the joy occurring in His Kingdom. Jesus is the Way through in our troubled times, and His joy keeps us connected to Him. Our whole being—body, soul, and spirit—works well together when connected to Him. Joy is evidence that God is near and we are near to Him.

You know what never gets old for me? Watching instructors in training get off the bus with bodies that feel like survival suits and five days later watching them get back on the bus wearing garments of praise. They often come feeling a little (or a lot) disconnected from God, themselves, and others, but they leave reconnected to lives overflowing with joy. They come feeling a little pooped and leave as party people!

People of God are party people.

In John 2:1-11, we read about Jesus' first miracle—the time He saved a party that was about to run out of wine. (In the Bible, wine represents joy and celebration.) When His mother, Mary, pointed out that they'd run out of wine, Jesus responded: "Woman, what does this have to do with me? My hour has not yet come." It doesn't appear that Jesus was planning on turning jugs of water into wine as his first miracle, but He heard the insistence in His mama's voice. Let's not forget, though: Jesus did only what He saw His Father doing. When Jesus went to the wedding, He probably wasn't thinking, *Tonight's the night!* He was waiting on the Father to tell Him what and when He should reveal His Father's Kingdom through His first miracle. But perhaps as His mama, Mary, looked at Him with expectant eyes, He caught a glimpse of His Father and heard something like *Now! It's time. Let's bring in our Kingdom by upgrading this party while pleasing your mama's heart.* To me, saving a wedding reception sounds like something a good God would do. I think He finds joy in our enjoyment of life.

Before Jesus saved the world, He saved a party.

Jesus' first miracle upgraded the joy in a joyful moment. Imagine then what good He can bring to those enduring what feels like a bad moment!

What a hurting world needs now is the love, joy, and peace of Jesus. This is our good work to do. We are here to show others the way to Jesus: "He said to them, 'Go into all the world and proclaim the gospel to the whole creation'" (Mark 16:15).

Let Joy Have the Last Word

C. S. Lewis said, "Joy is the serious business of heaven."[1] God is intent on filling us with what Jesus paid for us to have—joy! Our bodies give us a way to be about our Father's business of joy. We are here to go and tell others about the love of Jesus and the joy He brings.

Use your voice to speak what God is saying, use your eyes to see what He is doing, and use your body to go and do as He does. If what you desire is temporal and not connected to joy and confidence in God, submit that desire to the Lord. For a moment it will feel like suffering as the desire burns on the altar of your heart, but after the feeling of burning passes (similar to what you experience after doing that last squat), you will receive more joy. You'll be on the right track to staying free and setting others free while not losing your joy.

Our wellness doesn't match that of people who want to be well in body and mind but don't want God. They eat all the right things, think good thoughts, and reap the benefits. They treat their bodies like temples when really they're shrines to the self. They believe that if they live well enough, are good to others, and make good choices, they will have good lives and avoid pain and suffering. Those who don't want God get healthy to escape a world that's burning down, while the people of God get healthy so they can run back into the fire. With the joy of the Lord as their strength, they turn around and run back into the fire to help those who are burning with the same pain, showing them the way of escape. Jesus is the Way.

More than aiming to fill your body with plenty of water and whole foods, continually strive to fill your body with God's presence. Then go! Show and tell others about Jesus because you carry the presence of God in your body, which is the fullness of joy.

> You make known to me the path of life; in your presence there is fullness of joy; at your right hand are pleasures forevermore.
> PSALM 16:11

More than aiming to fill your body with plenty of water and whole foods, continually strive to fill your body with God's presence.

By doing the Metabolize portions of this book, you've been training your mind and your body to become a hospitable place for the Holy Spirit to rest. Continue to be a good host! Because the Holy Spirit has chosen to take up permanent residence in you, your body is host to the presence of heaven. Be agreeable to what the Holy Spirit wants to do. Tend to His needs. Ask Him what He would like to eat or drink, what He would like to do each day, or the sights He would like to see. Turn up the joy!

Good hosts of the Holy Spirit are ready and fully funded by God to throw good news parties wherever they go. They know that the sufferings of this world are transitory, their earthly bodies are temporary, and heaven is their eternal home. They want to please God's heart by stewarding well what they've been given (like their bodies). Their goal is to increase good, especially in difficult times, so others will see and choose God, and none will perish in their pain. People who run back into the fire to save others do not fear death or bodily decay, for no one can threaten to take away their home in heaven—the place they already live from filled with righteousness, peace, and joy.

It's been a couple of years since the passing of my mom and dad. For as much torment as they lived through here on earth, heaven got the final say. When they accepted Jesus as their Lord and Savior, they were saved. Like many Christians, they received salvation but missed out on transformation since they didn't know how to come to God to metabolize their pain. I know they are in heaven now, enjoying God, pain-free, lacking nothing and complete. My great cloud of witnesses got bigger, louder, and—considering how much my mom loved sparkly things—probably a whole lot blingier.

Keep Moving Out and Up

After Tammy spent five sweaty days completely immersing herself in the love of God and His people, she left the instructor training retreat feeling like a new person. Although she didn't lose a pound, her frozen shoulder, which had kept her from lifting her arm over her head, was completely healed. The stuff that had been stuck in her body moved out by faith! Tammy learned what it takes to embody her faith—to worship God with her whole self as she gave her whole self to God. The Holy Spirit put her on like a glove as she did and said things she never thought she could. Tammy worked out her salvation until she was transformed into someone new. Seven years later Tammy is still "revving"—getting free, staying free, and setting others free through fitness!

Friends, stay the course. Carry on the good work of working out your salvation. Remember and apply what you've learned in this book. If you get lost and find yourself navel-gazing about the hurt someone caused you or fixating on the number that measures your gravitational pull, remember who the real enemy is. Refer back to the stages in this book to figure out where you are in relationship to your pain and retrain yourself with some of the spiritual and physical practices needed to metabolize your pain.

When you feel pain or the tension of temptation and want to disconnect from God, giving yourself over to your momentarily misplaced desires and what the world says your body should look like, "re-member" yourself back to God. Reconnect yourself to the truth that you are no longer an orphan living in survival mode. You've been chosen and adopted into the family of God! You are a member of God's household with authority, rights, and privileges.

You now know what to do when stress, pain, and persecution come. Metabolize your pain! Let the Holy Spirit put you on like a glove. Get in your body and get with the Holy Spirit. Be still and breathe or go for a gentle walk or brisk run. By getting into your body, you will stir up the chemicals that fight off sickness and disease. Keep putting into practice everything you've learned in this book.

Reenter the Kingdom of God like the child you are. If you're tired, take a nap. If you're hungry, nourish yourself. Eat well so you can think, work, play, dance, and sing. And while you do these things, consider God's Word and let that Word speak. When you look in a mirror, see God seeing you and then reflect His image. When your smoke detector, your amygdala, sounds its alarm, don't freak out. Stay present in your body. Don't evacuate. Breathe. The Holy Spirit is inviting you to stay in the joy of heaven, a celebration where there is a table reserved for you. The enemy trembles at your joy, your peace, and your ability to sit down and eat.

God will never change His mind concerning you. You are God's good idea!

Never stop being and doing good with the body you've been given.

Metabolize

Mind

1. As you've worked through this book, in what ways have you begun to metabolize your pain to improve your health? Your joy?
2. When it comes to your body's health, what does it mean for you to have the joy of the Lord as your strength?
3. What will you do the next time you experience pain?

Mouth

Father, You are my joy! Thank You for my body. I rejoice in all it can do. Fill this body with Your presence and Your joy, which I want to be my strength! I want to host Your presence without end. Help me be a good host so I can go and tell others about You with the same joy You have given me. Thank You for saving all of me, including my body. I now declare that my body is good and that it belongs to You for goodness' sake. I will no longer worry more about the shape of my waistline than the condition of my heart. I know I am loved by You, a Good Father, and You have good work for me to do. Until I take my last breath and see You face-to-face, I give You my heart and now my body too.

Move

Let's celebrate! Take ten minutes to listen to this Be Still and Be Loved meditation: https://www.revelationwellness.org/tbr/still/. Sometime today, lace up your shoes, and move your body with the joy of the Lord as your strength: https://www.revelationwellness.org/tbr/move/.

ACKNOWLEDGMENTS

ALWAYS FIRST AND MOST, I acknowledge God: My Father. My Maker. My Husband when I didn't have one. I love You. Thank You for always being for me and with me. With You, Jesus, all things really are possible (Matthew 19:26). Every book idea comes from You, and this book's completion feels like Your miracle. Thank You for writing it through me and to the Holy Spirit for convincing me to sit my butt down to write when my mind was certain that I needed to clean the lint from my dryer first. You've taught me not to trust my feelings and to do hard things until they become easy. This book is Yours, Abba. Do with it as You wish. Then let's do it again soon! I love witnessing Your miracles.

This book would not have been written without the tens of thousands of bold, courageous, and beautiful Revelation Wellness students and instructors around the world. You are men and women of all ages, shapes, sizes, abilities, and beautiful God-colors who love God but have struggled to feel loved by Him and to walk in His ways—men and women who have cast off constraints and body shame. Thank you that, even though you didn't understand why God was calling you to put on workout clothes, get in your bodies, and meet with Him regarding the things that cause you pain, you did it anyway. Watching some of you show up to weeks of training, a little (or a lot) fractured, and then leave whole and more in love with God and ready to love people (especially the ones who are hard to love) encourages me. Your testimonies of how loving God and giving Him your bodies have changed you into new people are the reason I get up at the crack of dawn to begin the sometimes daunting task of staring down at a blank page to write. Some of your stories are woven into the pages of this book (though I have changed your names and identifying details). Although my body will fail me as I age and my wiggle won't be as juicy as it once was, I hope to leave you with many words, inspired by the Holy Spirit, to pass on to your children and their children's children, until a new standard has been raised and set for what it means to love God with our bodies and to be "fit."

Thank you for not just being hearers of the Word but doers of the Word and for knowing that all your doing comes from rest. Thank you for being humble, teachable, and healthy (but not perfect) disciples of Christ who subdue, have dominion, and multiply good by making healthy disciples of Christ. You are people who get free, stay free, and set others free! Revelation Wellness family, you are an extension of the dream for a family I never had growing up and are evidence that God knows our pain, hears our cries, and answers our prayers.

I couldn't have written this book without the support of the staff members and board of Revelation Wellness, the fifty-six men and women around the United States who lead and love like Jesus. You are some of my greatest teachers and God's refining tools, shaping and molding me into the image of Christ. You make work feel like play. God really is in a good mood, and you bring that mood into every Zoom room meeting or in-person filming, training, event, or retreat. Thank you for putting up with my need to throw confetti in the air everywhere we go and for cleaning up these holy messes in my wake.

We do hard things well, together. Let's keep beating the drum of health and wholeness—loving the fear, shame, and guilt out of people's bodies until earth looks like heaven and heaven is home to every soul Christ died to win! I've lost count of the times I've looked a staff or board member with tears in my eyes and said, "Can you believe we get to do this?"

Thank you to my board, who ask the big and hard questions of an ordinary girl like me. Working with you all is pure joy. A special thank you to chief officers Matt Golz and Tracy East for bringing order to my creative chaos and for carrying a heavy load with grace and ease. And to executive directors Fran Patoskie, Katrina Canfield, and Kristen Ulin: Thank you for being the cheerleaders and iron sharpeners you are to me, and for telling me no kindly and clearly when needed.

To the mission movers of Revelation Wellness, our financial partners who have given once or continually through the years, thank you! The afore acknowledged people wouldn't get to do what they do without you! Your generosity fuels the engine of this ministry, which breaks physical and spiritual chains of poverty. Wherever there are people feeling distant from God, hurting in body, heart, or mind, you send us, and we will go.

A special shout-out to Jess Connolly for writing the foreword to this book. Body freedom was your battle cry from the moment we met, and you haven't shrunk back one inch. You were one of the first students I was able to coach/ train without toning down my love for Jesus and the mission of Revelation Wellness. I have watched you, the student, become the teacher, charging the front lines of the body freedom battle. This godmother of freedom (a title you bestowed upon me that I joyfully accept) couldn't be prouder. I thank God for your middle-of-the-night email. (If you haven't read her book *Breaking Free from Body Shame*, do yourself a favor and get it now!)

Thank you to my writing coach, Nika Maples, for keeping me writing when all I had on the page was a mess of words with just a clear vision for who this book was for.

To Leah, Tammy, Dana, Carole, Renee, Krista, Jessica, Alyssa, Jodie, Sarah, Julie, Francie, and the entire sisterhood, your prayers have been powerful and effective for my family and the ministry of Revelation Wellness. Your friendship means the world to me.

Speaking of prayers: When I didn't have a literary agent, didn't have time to find a literary agent, and wouldn't even have known how to find one if I *did* have the time, I prayed: *God, please send someone to help me get this next book into the world.* Soon afterward I received an email from Tawny Johnson of Illuminate Agency, asking if I wanted to meet. God hears our prayers. Tawny, you have firmly and lovingly pushed me to the edge where my message has clarity and matches the passion and mission of Revelation Wellness. I look forward to finding out what immeasurably more messages are within me. Thanks for representing me like I am royalty.

To Kara, Jan, Kim, and the whole publishing team at Tyndale: I consider myself crazy blessed to publish another book with a reputable publishing firm that holds the Word of God in highest esteem. Kara, you are my girl! The fact that you don't just know about Revelation Wellness but *do* Revelation Wellness as part of your daily health plan and well-being is the best! You see me and get me, and you get what I've been called to do. Thank you for believing in me. Jan, I still thank God for Jill (a Revelation Wellness instructor) who handed you a spiral-bound, Xeroxed copy of my first manuscript, which turned into *The Wellness Revelation*. Thank you for continuing to take a risk on me in a field of health and wellness while the church is starting to get on board and see the need. I am honored to be a voice of Tyndale Refresh. (If you are still reading this book, all the way to the acknowledgments, it's because Kim—sweet, sweet Kim, my editor extraordinaire—made you want to keep reading.) Thank you for knowing my voice, honoring my voice, and making my voice better and clear. (And I think I finally understand how to work Track Changes. *Growth!*)

Jack and Sophia, thank you for standing by your little mama who is a whole lotta woman. I love you both with all of who God made me to be. You are God's greatest gifts to me, and you have taught me the most about how to heal; to humble myself, be wrong, say I was wrong, ask for forgiveness, ask what I can do better, and then be restored back into relationship with you. You've always been quick to forgive me, help me up, brush me off, and send me back on mission to do what God's called me to do. I'm so stupid blessed to be your mom. God knew what He was doing when He placed you in my womb. Revelation Wellness might be my ministry, but you two are my legacy.

Simon, my best friend: Twenty-five years ago, you casually told me, "You should write a book," and here we are three books, two kids, and a Stanley dog later. I love you more today than I did back then. Some days I feel like a schoolgirl crushing on a boy who thinks she's cute. But our wrinkles tell us another story. Our love story is one for the halls of faith. By God's grace we keep making it through better or worse. With our now-empty nest and extra time and energy to give each other, I look forward to the best of days ahead. Watching God restore the years the locusts ate makes our enemy rue the day he tried to mess with us. God wins! Thank you for believing in me and honoring marriage to the best of your ability even when you weren't sure what you believed in. You are a wonderful lover, provider, and protector of our family. Our children know God as a Father better because of your devotion to honor what is excellent, true, and praiseworthy.

ADVERSE CHILDHOOD EXPERIENCES (ACE) QUESTIONNAIRE

INSTRUCTIONS: Below is a list of ten categories of Adverse Childhood Experiences (ACEs).[1] Please place a checkmark next to each ACE category that you experienced prior to your eighteenth birthday. Then add up the number of ACE categories you experienced and put the total number at the bottom.

☐ Did a parent or other adult in the household often or very often swear at you, insult you, put you down, or humiliate you? Or act in a way that made you afraid that you might be physically hurt?

☐ Did a parent or other adult in the household often or very often push, grab, slap, or throw something at you? Or ever hit you so hard that you had marks or were injured?

☐ Did an adult or person at least five years older than you ever touch or fondle you or have you touch their body in a sexual way? Or attempt or actually have oral, anal, or vaginal intercourse with you?

☐ Did you often or very often feel that no one in your family loved you or thought you were important or special? Or your family didn't look out for each other, feel close to each other, or support each other?

☐ Did you often or very often feel that you didn't have enough to eat, had to wear dirty clothes, and had no one to protect you? Or your parents were too drunk or high to take care of you or take you to the doctor if needed?

☐ Was a biological parent ever lost to you through divorce, abandonment, or other reason?

☐ Was your mother or stepmother often or very often pushed, grabbed, slapped, or had something thrown at her? Or sometimes, often, or very often kicked, bitten, hit with a fist, or hit with something hard? Or ever repeatedly hit over at least a few minutes or threatened with a gun or knife?

☐ Did you live with anyone who was a problem drinker or alcoholic, or who used street drugs?

☐ Was a household member depressed or mentally ill, or did a household member attempt suicide?

☐ Did a household member go to prison?

Total: _____

MORE MOVEMENT LINKS

BELOW ARE MORE WAYS TO EXPLORE moving your body, without judgment, through RevWell TV. All videos have modifiers to help you move better while connecting your body back to God.

Follow the link below to access any of these workouts for free: revelationwellness.org/playlists/tbr-workout/.

1. Alisa's Cardio Intervals "Inherent Power"
2. Kara's Cardio Kickboxing "Trust the Trainer"
3. Courtney's Strength Training "A Tall Order"
4. Amia's Thirty-Minute Stretch "Precious Promises"
5. Demetria's Metabolic Strength "Taking New Ground"
6. Alisa's Strength Training "Yes in God"
7. Jerry's Cardio Intervals "Delighting in the Discipline"
8. Amia's Core Strength "Beyond Better"
9. Alisa's Cardio Strength "Knowing and Obeying"
10. Tammy's Flexibility and Mobility "Conformed, Called, and Glorified"
11. Torie's Kickboxing HIIT "Spiritual Identity"
12. Kara's Choreographed Strength "Fullness of Joy"
13. Alisa's Rev on the Mat "All Things Held Together"
14. Tammy's Cardio Strength "Training with Purpose"

15. Bri's Mobility and Stretch "Come Alive"
16. Alisa's Cardio Strength "Ask, Seek, Knock"
17. Demetria's Cardio/Strength Intervals "Confident Hope"
18. Michele's Rev on the Mat "The Heartbeat of the Father"
19. Sara's Choreography Mash-Up "God's Peace Is Our Peace"
20. Katrina's Strength Training "Choose Love Over Fear"

FOOD JOURNAL TEMPLATE

Date: _____   **Day:** _____

Verse of the Day: _____

_____

_____

Breakfast	Lunch	Dinner
🕐	🕐	🕐
Feelings/Thoughts:	*Feelings/Thoughts:*	*Feelings/Thoughts:*

Breakfast	Lunch	Dinner

Hunger Scale (circle one)

Before	*Before*	*Before*
1 2 3 4 5	1 2 3 4 5	1 2 3 4 5
After	*After*	*After*
1 2 3 4 5	1 2 3 4 5	1 2 3 4 5

Snacks: _____

Drinks: _____

Movement: _____

Quiet Time: Yes *or* No

How did I feel in my body today? _____

_____

_____

What is God teaching me? _____

_____

_____

_____

_____

This is a sample page from the Revelation Wellness food journal called *Not Your Average Food Journal*. Feel free to use as a template and make your own. The complete ninety-day journal is available from your favorite bookseller and includes more resources that are compatible with this book.

NOTES

INTRODUCTION: MOVING THE BAD OUT OF YOUR GOOD BODY

1. John J. Ratey, "Can Exercise Help Treat Anxiety?," Harvard Health Publishing website, October 24, 2018, https://www.health.harvard.edu/blog/can-exercise-help -treat-anxiety-2019102418096.

CHAPTER 1: THE FIRE OF YOUR DESIRE

1. "How Does Trauma Affect the Parasympathetic Nervous System?," Mental Health Systems, March 2, 2020, https://www.mhs-dbt.com/blog/parasympathetic-nervous -system-and-trauma.
2. Bessel A. van der Kolk, *The Body Keeps the Score: Brain, Mind, and Body in the Healing of Trauma* (New York: Penguin, 2014), 98–99.
3. Van der Kolk, *The Body Keeps the Score*, 98–99.
4. *Merriam-Webster's Collegiate Dictionary*, 11th ed. (2003), s.v. "desire."
5. Louise B. Miller, "What Causes Anger and How It Affects the Body," *Psychology Today*, July 16, 2020, https://www.psychologytoday.com/us/blog/the-mind-body -connection/202007/what-causes-anger-and-how-it-affects-the-body.
6. "Psychologists Find the Meaning of Aggression," The University of Texas at Austin, March 23, 2011, https://news.utexas.edu/2011/03/23/psychologists-find-the -meaning-of-aggression/.

CHAPTER 2: THE CALORIE BURN

1. Lexico, s.v. "metabolism," https://www.lexico.com/en/definition/metabolism (site discontinued).
2. Please note: Every theory is considered "fact" until it's disproved or until limitations are set. Currently, the theory of relativity (from which we get the idea that all matter has some form of energy) has not been disproved but is still considered theory.
3. "This Month in Physics History—May 1911: Rutherford and the Discovery of the Atomic Nucleus," *APS News* 15, no. 5 (May 2006): https://www.aps.org/publications /apsnews/200605/history.cfm.

CHAPTER 3: GOD'S TRANSFORMING FIRE

1. Bahman Zohuri, *Physics of Cryogenics: An Ultralow Temperature Phenomenon* (Amsterdam: Elsevier, 2017), 121.
2. Online Etymology Dictionary, s.v. "emotion," accessed September 7, 2022, https://www.etymonline.com/word/emotion.
3. Sebastian Schneegans and Gregor Schöner, "Dynamic Field Theory as a Framework for Understanding Embodied Cognition," in *Handbook of Cognitive Science: An Embodied Approach*, ed. Paco Calvo and Antoni Gomila (Amsterdam: Elsevier, 2009), 241–271.
4. Marjorie S. Miller, "Negative Mood Signals Body's Immune Response," The Penn State University press release, December 20, 2018, https://www.psu.edu/news/research/story/negative-mood-signals-bodys-immune-response/.

CHAPTER 4: GOD'S BURNING DESIRE FOR YOU

1. "The Water in You: Water and the Human Body," Water Science School, US Department of the Interior, May 22, 2019, https://www.usgs.gov/special-topics/water-science-school/science/water-you-water-and-human-body.

CHAPTER 5: PAIN AND THE EARLY BODY AND BRAIN

1. Vincent J. Felitti et al., "Relationship of Childhood Abuse and Household Dysfunction to Many of the Leading Causes of Death in Adults: The Adverse Childhood Experiences (ACE) Study," *American Journal of Preventive Medicine* 56, no. 6 (June 1, 2019): 774–786, https://psycnet.apa.org/record/2019-41272-005.
2. Donna Jackson Nakazawa, *Childhood Disrupted: How Your Biography Becomes Your Biology, and How You Can Heal* (New York: Atria, 2015), 14–15.
3. National Scientific Council on the Developing Child, (2005/2014), "Excessive Stress Disrupts the Architeture of the Developing Brain: Working Paper 3," January 2014, 3, https://developingchild.harvard.edu/wp-content/uploads/2005/05/Stress_Disrupts_Architecture_Developing_Brain-1.pdf.
4. Denise Schipani, "Here's How Stress and Inflammation Are Linked," *Everyday Health*, October 16, 2018, https://www.everydayhealth.com/wellness/united-states-of-stress/link-between-stress-inflammation/.
5. Yun-Zi Liu, Yun-Xia Wang, and Chun-Lei Jiang, "Inflammation: The Common Pathway of Stress-Related Diseases," *Frontiers in Human Neuroscience* 11 (June 20, 2017), https://www.frontiersin.org/articles/10.3389/fnhum.2017.00316.
6. Gabor Maté, *When the Body Says No* (Hoboken, NJ: John Wiley & Sons, 2003), 3. See also Clayton E. Tucker-Ladd, *Psychological Self-Help* (self-pub. Liviant, 1996), https://www.psychologicalselfhelp.org/Chapter7/chap7_107.html.
7. Henri J. M. Nouwen, *The Life of the Beloved: Spiritual Living in a Secular World* (New York: Crossroad, 1992), 75.

CHAPTER 6: HOW PAIN CHANGES YOUR BODY AND BRAIN

1. SAMHSA's Trauma and Justice Strategic Initiative, "SAMHSA's Concept of Trauma and Guide for a Trauma-Informed Approach," July 7, 2014, https://store.samhsa.gov/sites/default/files/d7/priv/sma14-4884.pdf.
2. Elyssa Barbash, "Different Types of Trauma: Small 't' versus Large 'T,'" *Psychology Today*, March 13, 2017, https://www.psychologytoday.com/us/blog/trauma-and-hope/201703/different-types-trauma-small-t-versus-large-t.

3. "The Long-Term Effects of Trauma and How to Deal with It," Northpoint Recovery, February 28, 2017, https://www.northpointrecovery.com/blog/long-term-effects -trauma-deal/.

4. "Everything You Need to Know about Stress," Healthline, updated February 25, 2020, https://www.healthline.com/health/stress.

CHAPTER 7: WHERE PAIN GOES IN YOUR BRAIN

1. Jacob Tindle and Prasanna Tadi, *Neuroanatomy, Parasympathetic Nervous System* (Treasure Island, FL: StatPearls Publishing), 2022, https://www.ncbi.nlm.nih.gov /books/NBK553141/.

2. Peter A. Levine, *Waking the Tiger: Healing Trauma* (Berkeley, CA: North Atlantic Books, 1997), 19–21.

3. *Merriam-Webster's Collegiate Dictionary*, 11th ed. (2003), s.v. "perspective."

4. "Understanding the Teen Brain," University of Rochester Medical Center, Health Encyclopedia, https://www.urmc.rochester.edu/encyclopedia/content.aspx?Content TypeID=1&ContentID=305.

5. Bessel A. van der Kolk, *The Body Keeps the Score: Brain, Mind, and Body in the Healing of Trauma* (New York: Penguin, 2014), 60–62.

6. "Amygdala Hijack: When Emotion Takes Over," Healthline, updated September 17, 2021, https://www.healthline.com/health/stress/amygdala-hijack.

7. "The Limbic System," The University of Queensland Australia, Queensland Brain Institute, https://qbi.uq.edu.au/brain/brain-anatomy/limbic-system.

8. Van der Kolk, *The Body Keeps the Score*, 62.

9. Bill Conklin, "The Role of the Brain in Happiness," In the Face of Adversity, *Psychology Today*, February 19, 2013, https://www.psychologytoday.com/us/blog/in-the-face-adversity/201302/the-role-the-brain-in-happiness.

10. "Caroline Leaf Quotes," Goodreads, accessed September 7, 2022, https://www .goodreads.com/quotes/1205028-our-brains-are-made-for-love-not-fear-not -performance.

CHAPTER 8: TENSION VS. PAIN

1. *Strong's Hebrew Lexicon* H3533, s.v. "kabas."

2. *Strong's Hebrew Lexicon* H7287, s.v. "rada."

3. *Merriam-Webster's Collegiate Dictionary*, 11th ed. (2003), s.v. "tension."

CHAPTER 9: FEELING YOUR FEELINGS

1. Clinical psychologist Paul Ekman is credited with identifying six core emotions; based on universal facial expressions, he later identified a seventh (contempt).

2. Andrea Brandt, "To Heal from Trauma, You Have to Feel Your Feelings," *Psychology Today*, October 2, 2019, https://www.psychologytoday.com/blog/mindful-anger /201910/heal-trauma-you-have-feel-your-feelings.

3. "How Do Thoughts and Emotions Affect Health?" University of Minnesota, Earl E. Bakken Center for Spirituality and Healing, 2016, https://www.takingcharge.csh .umn.edu/how-do-thoughts-and-emotions-affect-health.

4. Carroll E. Izard, "Emotion Theory and Research: Highlights, Unanswered Questions, and Emerging Issues," *Annual Review of Psychology* 60 (2009): 1–25, https://www .ncbi.nlm.nih.gov/pmc/articles/PMC2723854/.

5. Stuart W. G. Derbyshire and John C. Bockmann, "Reconsidering Fetal Pain," *Journal of Medical Ethics* 46, no. 1 (2020): 3–6, https://jme.bmj.com/content/46/1/3.

CHAPTER 10: EXTINGUISHING PAIN

1. James J. DiNicolantonio, James H. O'Keefe, William L. Wilson, "Sugar Addiction: Is It Real? A Narrative Review," *British Journal of Sports Medicine* 52, no. 14 (July 2018): 910–913.
2. Anna Lembke, *Dopamine Nation* (New York: Dutton, 2021), 53.
3. While carbohydrates are the body's primary source of glucose, proteins and fats can also be converted to glycogen, though this happens indirectly and when a person fasts or goes on a no-carb diet. The body is smart; it will find a way to get glycogen. See Claire Fromentin et al., "Dietary Proteins Contribute Little to Glucose Production, Even under Optimal Gluconeogenic Conditions in Healthy Humans," *Diabetes* 62, no. 5 (May 2013): 1435–1442, https://pubmed.ncbi.nlm.nih.gov/23274906/; Derek Bryan, "Can Fats Be Turned into Glycogen for Muscle?" SFGATE, December 27, 2018, https://healthyeating.sfgate.com/can-fats-turned-glycogen-muscle-11127 .html.
4. Roma Pahwa, Amandeep Goyal, and Ishwaral Jialal, *Chronic Inflammation* (Treasure Island, FL: StatPearls Publishing, 2022), https://www.ncbi.nlm.nih.gov/books /NBK493173/.
5. C. P. Chong et al., "Habitual Sugar Intake and Cognitive Impairment among Multiethnic Malaysian Older Adults," *Clinical Interventions in Aging* 14 (July 22, 2019): 1331–1342, https://www.ncbi.nlm.nih.gov/pmc/articles/PMC6662517/; Scott Edwards, "Sugar and the Brain," Harvard Medical School, spring 2016, https://hms.harvard.edu/news-events/publications-archive/brain/sugar-brain.
6. "Added Sugar," Harvard T. H. Chan School of Public Health, https://www.hsph .harvard.edu/nutritionsource/carbohydrates/added-sugar-in-the-diet/.
7. Yu Shang et al., "Noninvasive Optical Characterization of Muscle Blood Flow, Oxygenation, and Metabolism in Women with Fibromyalgia," *Arthritis Research and Therapy* 14, no. 6 (November 1, 2012): R236, https://pubmed.ncbi.nlm.nih .gov/23116302/.
8. Aundi Kolber, *Try Softer: A Fresh Approach to Move Us out of Anxiety, Stress, and Survival Mode—and into a Life of Connection and Joy* (Carol Stream, IL: Tyndale, 2020).
9. "My Stroke of Insight," TED Talk by Dr. Jill Bolte Taylor, posted March 13, 2008, https://www.youtube.com/watch?v=UyyjU8fzEYU.

CHAPTER 11: KINDNESS AND SELF-COMPASSION

1. "Kindness Health Facts," randomactsofkindness.org, https://www.dartmouth.edu /wellness/emotional/rakhealthfacts.pdf; "The Science of Kindness," Cedars-Sinai, February 13, 2019, https://www.cedars-sinai.org/blog/science-of-kindness.html.
2. Paul Gilbert, *The Compassionate Mind* (Oakland, CA: New Harbinger Press, 2009), 44.
3. "Empathy Builds Connections," University of Kentucky Cooperative Extension, 2020, https://powell.ca.uky.edu/files/empathybuildsconnection.pdf.
4. "The Science of Kindness," Cedars-Sinai blog, https://www.cedars-sinai.org/blog /science-of-kindness.html.

CHAPTER 12: MINDFULNESS AND MINDFUL MOVEMENT

1. Bessel A. van der Kolk, *The Body Keeps The Score: Brain, Mind, and Body in the Healing of Trauma* (New York: Penguin, 2014), 96–97.

2. Michael Winnick, "Putting a Finger on Our Phone Obsession," dscout, June 16, 2016, https://dscout.com/people-nerds/mobile-touches.

3. Erica Cirino, "Chewing Your Food: Is 32 Really the Magic Number?" Healthline, updated March 19, 2020, https://www.healthline.com/health/how-many-times-should-you-chew-your-food.

4. Sue McGreevey, "Eight Weeks to a Better Brain," *Harvard Gazette*, January 21, 2011, https://news.harvard.edu/gazette/story/2011/01/eight-weeks-to-a-better-brain.

5. K. Carrière et al., "Mindfulness-Based Interventions for Weight Loss: A Systematic Review and Meta-analysis," *Obesity Reviews* 19, no. 2 (February 2018): 164–77, https://pubmed.ncbi.nlm.nih.gov/29076610/.

6. Michaela C. Pascoe et al., "Mindfulness Mediates the Physiological Markers of Stress: Systematic Review and Meta-Analysis," *Journal of Psychiatric Research* 95 (December 2017): 156–178, https://pubmed.ncbi.nlm.nih.gov/28863392/.

7. Jennifer Daubenmier et al., "Mindfulness Intervention for Stress Eating to Reduce Cortisol and Abdominal Fat among Overweight and Obese Women: An Exploratory Randomized Controlled Study," *Journal of Obesity* (October 2011): https://www.hindawi.com/journals/jobe/2011/651936/.

8. Matthew Thorpe and Rachael Link, "12 Science-Based Benefits of Meditation," Healthline, updated October 27, 2020, https://www.healthline.com/nutrition/12-benefits-of-meditation.

9. Michelle W. Voss et al., "Bridging Animal and Human Models of Exercise-Induced Brain Plasticity," *Trends in Cognitive Sciences* 17, no. 10 (October 2013): 525–544, https://www.ncbi.nlm.nih.gov/pmc/articles/PMC4565723/.

CHAPTER 13: HUMILITY, NOT HUMILIATION

1. M. G. Easton, *Easton's Bible Dictionary*, s.v. "humility," accessed September 7, 2020, https://www.htmlbible.com/kjv30/easton/east1845.htm.

2. Elisabeth Elliot, *Discipline: The Glad Surrender* (Grand Rapids: Revell, 2006), 44.

CHAPTER 14: HELP! A FOUR-LETTER WORD

1. Jayne Leonard, "What Is Learned Helplessness?" Medical News Today, updated September 1, 2022, https://www.medicalnewstoday.com/articles/325355.

2. "Average Time Spent Daily on Social Media (Latest 2022 Data)," BroadbandSearch (blog), accessed October 19, 2022, https://www.broadbandsearch.net/blog/average-daily-time-on-social-media.

3. Curt P. Richter, "On the Phenomenon of Sudden Death in Animals and Man," *Psychosomatic Medicine* 19, no. 3 (May 1957): 191–198.

CHAPTER 15: KEEP GOING; IT'S ONLY A TEST

1. *Strong's Hebrew Lexicon* H5065, s.v. "nāḡaś," accessed September 7, 2022, https://www.blueletterbible.org/lexicon/h5065/kjv/wlc/0-1/.

2. *Strong's Greek Lexicon* G3101, s.v. "mathētēs," accessed September 7, 2022, https://www.blueletterbible.org/lexicon/g3101/kjv/tr/0-1/.

CHAPTER 16: WORKING FROM REST

1. Kirsten Nunez and Karen Lamoreux, "What Is the Purpose of Sleep?" Healthline, July 20, 2020, https://www.healthline.com/health/why-do-we-sleep.
2. "Sleep and Sleep Disorders: Data and Statistics," Centers for Disease Control and Prevention, reviewed September 12, 2022, https://www.cdc.gov/sleep/data_statistics.html.
3. George A. Timmons et al., "The Circadian Clock Protein BMAL1 Acts as a Metabolic Sensor In Macrophages to Control the Production of Pro IL-1β," *Frontiers in Immunology* 12 (November 9, 2021), https://pubmed.ncbi.nlm.nih.gov/34858390/.
4. David S. Black et al., "Mindfulness Meditation and Improvement in Sleep Quality and Daytime Impairment among Older Adults with Sleep Disturbances," *JAMA Internal Medicine* 175, no. 4 (April 1, 2015): 494–501, https://www.ncbi.nlm.nih.gov/pmc/articles/PMC4407465/.
5. Sarah Jackson, "Google CEO Sundar Pichai Says He uses NSDR, or 'Non-Sleep Deep Rest' to Unwind. Here Is What It Is and How It Works," *Business Insider*, March 5, 2022, https://www.businessinsider.com/google-ceo-sundar-pichai-non-sleep-deep-rest-nsdr-relax-2022-3.
6. Mark Buchanan, *The Holy Wild: Trusting in the Character of God* (Colorado Springs, CO: Multnomah, 2003), 26.

CHAPTER 18: YOUR NEW REALITY

1. "Dr. Quantum—Double Slit Experiment," YouTube, December 10, 2010, https://www.youtube.com/watch?v=Q1YqgPAtzho.
2. Jim Al-Khalili, *Quantum: A Guide for the Perplexed* (London: Orion, 2012), introduction; Daisy Dobrijevic, "The Double-Slit Experiment: Is Light a Wave or a Particle?" Space.com, March 23, 2022, https://www.space.com/double-slit-experiment-light-wave-or-particle.
3. Max Planck, *The New Science*, as quoted by Goodreads, https://www.goodreads.com/quotes/7819522-as-a-man-who-has-devoted-his-whole-life-to.
4. Dallas Willard, *The Divine Conspiracy: Rediscovering Our Hidden Life in God* (New York: HarperCollins, 2014), 25.
5. Weizmann Institute of Science, "Quantum Theory Demonstrated Observation Affects Reality," *Science Daily*, February 27, 1998, https://www.sciencedaily.com/releases/1998/02/980227055013.htm.

CHAPTER 19: FORGIVENESS AND THE PARTY POOPERS

1. Johns Hopkins Medicine, "Forgiveness: Your Health Depends on It," https://www.hopkinsmedicine.org/health/wellness-and-prevention/forgiveness-your-health-depends-on-it.
2. Strong's Greek Lexicon G0863, s.v. "aphiēmi," accessed September 3, 2022, https://www.blueletterbible.org/lexicon/g863/kjv/tr/0-1/.
3. Ciro Conversano et al., "Optimism and Its Impact on Mental and Physical Well-Being," *Clinical Practice and Epidemiology in Mental Health* 6 (2010): 25–29, https://www.ncbi.nlm.nih.gov/pmc/articles/PMC2894461.

CHAPTER 20: TELLING YOURSELF THE TRUTH

1. Joanne V. Wood, W. Q. Elaine Perunovic, and John W. Lee, "Positive Self-Statements: Power for Some, Peril for Others," *Psychological Science* 20, no. 7 (July 2009): 860–866, https://pubmed.ncbi.nlm.nih.gov/19493324/.

CHAPTER 22: HAVE A VISION FOR YOUR FUTURE

1. Tracy C. Ekeocha, "The Effects of Visualization and Guided Imagery in Sports Performance" (master's thesis, Texas State University, May 2015), 11 https://digital .library.txstate.edu/bitstream/handle/10877/5548/EKEOCHA-THESIS-2015.pdf.

CHAPTER 23: WORDS CREATE YOUR WORLD

1. Masaru Emoto, *The Hidden Messages in Water* (New York: Atria, 2005).
2. Andrew Newberg and Mark Robert Waldman, *Words Can Change Your Brain: 12 Conversation Strategies to Build Trust, Resolve Conflict, and Increase Intimacy* (New York: Plume, 2013), 24.

CHAPTER 24: CELEBRATE!

1. C. S. Lewis, *Letters to Malcolm, Chiefly on Prayer* (New York: HarperOne, 1964), letter 17.

ADVERSE CHILDHOOD EXPERIENCES (ACE) QUESTIONNAIRE

1. James A. Reavis et al., "Adverse Childhood Experiences and Adult Criminality: How Long Must We Live before We Possess Our Own Lives?" *Permanente Journal* 17, no. 2 (spring 2013): 44–48. See also Centers for Disease Control and Prevention, "About the CDC-Kaiser ACE Study," https://www.cdc.gov/violenceprevention /aces/about.html.

ABOUT THE AUTHOR

ALISA KEETON is a wholehearted pursuer of God's love in heart, mind, soul, and strength. A fitness professional for over thirty years, she is the founder of Revelation Wellness, a nonprofit ministry that uses physical and mental health practices to spread the gospel by inviting participants to become integrated and whole through biblical teachings, online events, productions, and in-person retreat experiences. Alisa is the author of *The Wellness Revelation* and *Heir to the Crown* and hosts the popular *Revelation Wellness* podcast with over seven million downloads. Alisa lives in Phoenix with her husband, Simon, and they have two children, Jack and Sophia. As a family, they are on a mission to change the world with the kind and courageous love of God.

Continue your good body journey with Alisa Keeton as she encourages you to love God, get healthy, and serve others!

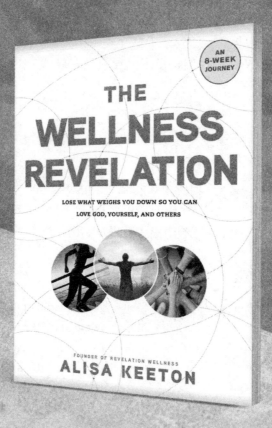

The Wellness Revelation will change the way you see yourself and the way you live your life. Alisa Keeton, founder of Revelation Wellness, will provide you with the tools you need to feel strong and spread the gospel with courage, confidence, kindness, and freedom.

It's time to make a change from the inside out.

Available wherever books are sold.

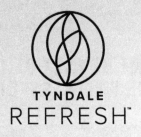

TYNDALE
REFRESH™

Think Well. Live Well. Be Well.

Experience the flourishing of your mind, body, and soul with Tyndale Refresh.

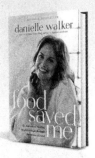
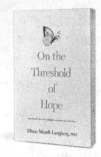
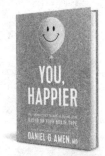

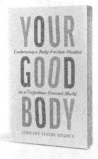
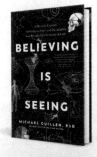
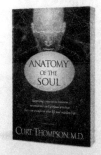

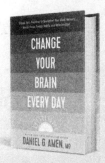
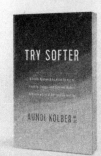
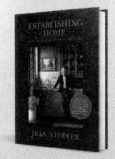

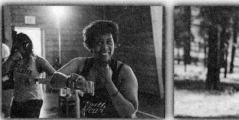
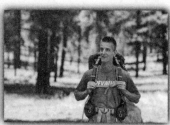